DATE DUE

DEC 9 1998	
GAYLORD	PRINTED IN U.S.A.

Motor Disorder in Psychiatry

Motor Disorder in Psychiatry
Towards a Neurological Psychiatry

DANIEL ROGERS

Burden Neurological Hospital, Bristol, UK

JOHN WILEY & SONS

Chichester · New York · Brisbane · Toronto · Singapore

RC
376.5
.R64
1992

Other Wiley Editorial Offices

John Wiley & Sons, Inc., 605 Third Avenue,
New York, NY 10158-0012, USA

Jacaranda Wiley Ltd, G.P.O. Box 859, Brisbane,
Queensland 4001, Australia

John Wiley & Sons (Canada) Ltd, 22 Worcester Road,
Rexdale, Ontario M9W 1L1, Canada

John Wiley & Sons (SEA) Pte Ltd, 37 Jalan Pemimpin #05-04,
Block B, Union Industrial Building, Singapore 2057

Library of Congress Cataloging-in-Publication Data

Rogers, Daniel M., 1909–
    Motor disorder in psychiatry : towards a neurological psychiatry
Daniel Rogers.
        p.   cm.
    Includes bibliographical references and index.
    ISBN 0 471 93616 2
    1. Psychomotor disorders.   2. Movement disorders.   I. Title.
    [DNLM: 1. Mental Disorders—complications.   2. Psychomotor
Disorders—complications.   WM 197 R725m]
    RC376.5.R64   1992
    616.8'4—dc20
    DNLM/DLC
    for Library of Congress   92-23748 CIP

British Library Cataloguing in Publication Data

A catalogue record for this book is available from the British Library

ISBN 0 471 93616 2

Typeset in 10/12pt Garamond by Mathematical Composition Setters Ltd, Salisbury
Printed and bound in Great Britain by Biddles Ltd, Guildford, Surrey

This book is dedicated to Dr Richard Hunter, the *fons et origo* of its ideas.

Contents

Preface

This book should also be dedicated to my mother-in-law. During my elective period as a medical student, I decided to investigate why there were such radically differing views on the nature of schizophrenia. My mother-in-law suggested that it would help to actually see some patients with the condition and arranged this through a psychiatrist to whom she was teaching French at evening classes, and who worked in the local psychiatric hospital. This was my introduction to Friern Hospital in North London. There I heard about one of the consultants who did not allow a diagnosis of schizophrenia in any of his patients. I obviously had to meet him and arranged to attend one of his ward rounds.

I remember vividly the sight, as I poked my head round the door, of Dr Richard Hunter, surrounded by his team, intently studying a patient in catatonic stupor. The scene looked like an illustration from a nineteenth-century psychiatric text-book. Richard Hunter then took me round the back wards of the hospital, filled with patients with a case-note diagnosis of schizophrenias which he considered as undiagnosed neurological illness. This was indeed a nineteenth-century view, so different from the currently orthodox view of schizophrenia. I later used the two views of a 'Necker cube' as an analogy for these two radically different views. Over the next 48 hours my view of the psychiatric Necker cube switched. The contrast between the two views was most obvious for motor disorder. This book was the result.

The first chapter describes how ideas on motor disorder in psychiatry developed, over the last 100 years, to the still currently orthodox position that psychiatric motor disorder is radically distinct from neurological motor disorder and that its cerebral basis is not essential to understanding it. The second chapter develops the same theme considering specifically extrapyramidal disorder and catatonia. Chapters 3, 4 and 5 consider the motor disorders of schizophrenia, affective disorder, obsessive–compulsive disorder, hysteria and mental handicap. Chapter 6 considers the contribution of medication to this motor disorder and the possible interaction between drug and disease induced motor disorder. Chapters 7 and 8 consider disturbances of posture, tone, voluntary motor performance, activity, abnormal movements and speech production found in psychiatric disorder. This is followed by four rating scales to assess motor disorder in psychiatric illness and an extensive list of references.

The thesis of this book is that motor disorder in psychiatry can be understood in terms of cerebral dysfunction, that there is no essential difference between motor disorder found in psychiatric and neurological disorders, and that a neurological approach to psychiatry is valid and worthwhile.

Preface

Acknowledgements

To Dr Michael Trimble of the National Hospital, Queen Square, for encouraging me to write the book and to Mrs Mary Raymond-Way for her generous support during my time at Queen Square.

1 Motor Disorder in Psychiatry and Neurology—The Necker Cube Phenomenon

A CURIOUS CHANGE

A curious thing happened in psychiatry at the end of the last century. Up till then psychiatry was becoming more and more securely brain-based. Consider the following quotations:

> Insanity being a disease, and that disease being an affection of the brain, it can therefore only be studied in a proper manner from the medical point of view (Griesinger 1845).

> So far as the phenomena of deranged mind reach, the battle has been won and the victory is complete; no one whose opinion is of any value pretends now that they are any thing more than the deranged functions of the supreme nervous centres of the body (Maudsley 1873).

The first quotation is from Wilhelm Griesinger's textbook of psychiatry (Griesinger 1845). Griesinger (1817–1868) was professor of psychiatry in Berlin at a time when Germany was pre-eminent in the field of psychiatry. For Griesinger, psychiatry and neuropathology were not merely two closely related fields but one field in which only one language was spoken and the same laws ruled. The second quotation is from Henry Maudsley's book *Mind and Body* (Maudsley 1873). Maudsley (1835–1918) was one of the most forward-looking English psychiatrists of his time. He left a legacy after his death in 1918 to found a neuropsychiatric hospital based on the ideas he developed in this book. The Maudsley hospital became England's premier psychiatric hospital.

For Griesinger and Maudsley, it was obvious that psychiatric disorder was synonymous with brain disorder. They saw this as the natural consequence of increasing understanding of brain function and the scientific basis of medicine. They recognised the limitations of their knowledge but looked forward to the inevitable further increase in knowledge of brain function and dysfunction, making greater and greater contributions to the understanding of psychiatric disorder.

They hardly imagined that interest in a brain-based approach to psychiatric disorder was shortly to diminish considerably and not resurface as a major force for some 100 years. Starting in the last decade of the nineteenth century, and for the first two-thirds of this century, a different approach to psychiatric disorder took centre stage—the investigation of abnormal mental states divorced from cerebral function.

This is well illustrated in Figure 1, which is taken from a monograph (Jelliffe 1932) on the eye movement disorder known as oculogyric crisis. It is still the best monograph on the subject. The author, Smith Ely Jelliffe, knew all about neurology. He was professor of diseases of the mind and nervous system at New York and co-author of one of the major textbooks of neurology and psychiatry of its time. His clinical descriptions of oculogyric crisis have not been surpassed. However, what he felt was new and exciting in trying to make sense of psychiatric disorder, and for that matter a lot of neurological disorder, was what he drew in his illustration—the possibility of exploring and mapping out the mind, just as neurologists were successfully exploring and mapping out the brain.

Smith Ely Jelliffe provides a very useful insight into the radical difference between this approach and that of Griesinger and Maudsley. For Jelliffe, it was the psychological meaning of motor disorder that was interesting and important: 'one understands bodily behaviour, if one understands its psychic meaning'. This was a common view at the time, but most authors confined this psychological approach to psychiatric disorders. Jelliffe, however, was entirely logical in applying the new approach. Since it was a conceptual approach aimed at attaching meaning to clinical phenomena it was as valid in neurological disorders, whose brain basis was known, as in psychiatric disorders, whose brain basis still awaited discovery. In different papers (Jelliffe 1927, 1940), he suggested, for example, that the flexed posture of the parkinsonian patient could be understood as repressed sadism and the drooling saliva of the post-encephalitic as 'displaced' seminal emission.

Such views did not gain widespread acceptance for neurological movement disorders, but for other movement disorders not firmly in the neurological fold, such as tics, psychological explanations were commonplace among neurologists as well as psychiatrists:

> No feature is more prominent in tic than its irresistibility. The strain of holding the movement back is as great as the relief in letting go . . . The element of compulsion links the condition intimately to the vast group of obsessions and fixed ideas . . . Behind all tic phenomena lies a psychical predisposition . . . A varying degree of mental infantilism . . . stigmatises the tiqueur; in the language of psychoanalysis, he is narcissistically fixed (Wilson 1927).

The gulf between what Oliver Sacks has called 'soulless neurology' and 'bodiless psychology' could not be wider. It is a conceptual divide and is thus unbridgeable. This was well appreciated by Bernard Hart, in his presidential address to the psychiatry section of the Royal Society of Medicine (Hart 1932) in the same year that Smith Ely Jelliffe's monograph appeared:

> Mental disorder is being attacked along a number of different avenues, which fall into two broad groups, on the one hand the psychological and on the other, what we will term the physiological . . . This second group . . . all follow the road of objective science . . . The psychological group follows a road which is radically different, in that it seeks to construct causal explanations out of the stuff of subjective experience . . . The psychologist can claim that his method . . . has at the present time indubitably achieved greater success than any other method (Hart 1932).

Hart again was no stranger to neurology. He was psychiatric consultant to the National Hospital for Nervous Diseases, Queen Square, in London, England's premier neurological hospital, and published papers in the neurological journal *Brain*. In the above quotation, he makes two important points:

- The two different views of psychiatric disorder, the brain-based scientific and the psychological non-scientific, are radically distinct.
- When he was writing in 1932, the psychological approach was the one he most favoured and felt likely to succeed.

This almost universal acceptance of the psychological approach during this period is important to appreciate today, as it was then that the foundations of contemporary psychiatry were being laid. For example, it was at this time that Aubrey Lewis, later to become the doyen of British psychiatry, was preparing the groundwork for our current understanding of depression. His acceptance of the new psychological approach was somewhat ambivalent; he called it legitimate but suggested that a pathophysiological approach would eventually be more fruitful. This ambivalence allowed him in the same paper, (Lewis 1934a), to castigate Karl Kleist, one of the few contemporary psychiatrists who had not embraced the new psychological approach, for being 'under the influence of biological tendencies', while at the same time declaring his faith in the biological conception of psychiatric disorder.

In order to resolve this ambivalent position, Lewis tried like many others then and later, to bridge the unbridgeable—the conceptual system exemplified in Figure 1 and one based on the brain. A full understanding of the close affinities between schizophrenia and severe chorea, for example, could only be reached from a synthesis of the psychological and pathophysiological approaches (Lewis & Minski 1935). Lewis argued as follows. He started from the apparently unexceptionable argument that it was impossible to separate sharply disturbance of function referable to structural damage from what was still best interpreted only in terms of function. He then maintained that this was equivalent to the division between physiological and psychological, and concluded that the only way forward was a synthesis between the two approaches. The second step in this argument, however, was flawed as it hinged on the ambivalent meaning of the word 'functions' which needs closer analysis, like its partner in crime 'organic'.

ORGANIC AND FUNCTIONAL

The dichotomy between organic and functional is not a simple one. Both terms, 'organic' and 'functional', have at least two distinct meanings. 'Organic' can mean anatomical or structural, or it can mean physical in origin. 'Functional' can mean physiological or it can mean mental in origin. There are, in fact, two distinct dichotomies denoted by the same antonyms, organic and functional.

The dichotomy between anatomical and physiological, or structural and functional, is a purely descriptive one, made between two complementary biological aspects of an organ or organism. When applied to pathology, it separates cases where there is recognisable macroscopic or microscopic change with currently available imaging techniques from cases where there is not. The dichotomy between physical and mental origin, however, is an aetiological one, made within a particular philosophical framework or paradigm, that of mind–body dualism. According to this paradigm, disorder of either body or mind is capable of causing illness in the organism.

The two dichotomies are clearly independent as well as distinct. Their terms, 'organic' and 'functional', are the only thing they have in common. For example, when a brain disorder is described as 'organic' it can mean a structural disorder, as opposed to a biochemical one, or simply that it is physical in origin. If an illness is described as 'functional', it can mean that no recognisable pathological change can be found or that it is thought to result from disorder of the mind. The two issues, presence of recognisable pathological change, and physical or mental origin, are completely separable and bear no necessary relation to each other.

There might, in practice, be reluctance to attribute a mental origin to a structural brain disorder but, logically, this is no more unlikely than a mental origin for non-structural disorder, which causes less qualms. Both structural and non-structural disorders of the brain are necessarily physical. The difficulties involved in mental causes for either apply equally to both. This problem is a philosophical one; type of pathology is not. Biochemical or electrical is not the same as mental.

Consider the following two statements:

- Depression in Parkinson's disease may result from a putative neurophysiological dysfunction or from a psychological reaction to the burden of the physical symptoms.
- Today it is either raining or it is Wednesday.

These two statements are equivalent. They contain the same logical flaw. The flaw is not so obvious in the first statement, but it is equally severe. The apparent alternatives offered are not true alternatives—they are not mutually exclusive. There are not two kinds of depression in Parkinson's disease but two ways of making sense of it.

The confusion that can result from not distinguishing between the two separate dichotomies described above is exemplified in the differentiation of organic from functional psychoses. Theoretically, for the historical reasons described in the last section, the difference between these is their presumed physical or mental origin but, in practice, it hinges on the presence or absence of recognised cerebral disorder. Although completely separate issues, the use of the ambivalent terms, 'organic' and 'functional', allows the distinction to be blurred, and paradox is produced.

The brain disorder of psychotic illnesses classified as 'functional' has been extensively studied but it is a study that can never bear fruit. When, in particular cases, brain disorder is established, these are no longer considered functional psychoses; not because those particular cases have been shown not to proceed from a mental origin, but because brain disorder has been established. This is sophistry whose only aim is to preserve the position in which psychiatry found itself at the beginning of this century. Its result is that research into the brain basis of functional psychosis is self-defeating; by definition it can never be discovered.

Accepting psychoses associated with known cerebral disorder as equivalent to those in which cerebral disorder is presumed but not established, is arguably the single most important step forward in research in this field. If we said 'structural' or 'physical' in origin, instead of 'organic', and 'non-structural' or 'mental' in origin, instead of 'functional', this step would be inevitable.

ONE MAN'S SCHIZOPHRENIA IS ANOTHER MAN'S ENCEPHALITIS

In 1917 the pandemic of encephalitis lethargica started sweeping across Asia and then Europe and America. It is remembered for its high mortality and the production, in a high proportion of its survivors, of post-encephalitic parkinsonism. It is possible that if it had started a generation before, present day psychiatry might be very different. As well as parkinsonism it produced in its victims every known psychiatric symptom and syndrome. Because of this, Constantin von Economo, in his monograph on the encephalitis which now bears his name (Economo 1931), suggested that psychiatry would never be the same again. The epidemic, however, had relatively little impact on psychiatry because, by the time it struck, psychiatry was more interested in psychology than neurology.

Eugene Bleuler launched the diagnosis of schizophrenia in his 1911 monograph (Bleuler 1911). At this time, he completely embraced the psychological ideas of Sigmund Freud and used these to interpret all its symptoms and signs. Even then, however, his approach was equivocal since he felt that a complete understanding of schizophrenia was not possible without considering the brain. He subsequently drew further and further away from a psychological approach (Steck 1943) and in the last edition of his textbook of psychiatry, published in 1937, accepted that acute cases of schizophrenia and encephalitis lethargica were indistinguishable, and that in chronic cases the distinction rested on the fact that, in his disease, mental symptoms were more prominent than motor, while, in von Economo's, motor symptoms were more prominent than mental (Hunter & Macalpine (1974, p. 227).

The psychological bandwagon once launched, however, kept rolling. Schizophrenia was the province of psychiatrists and encephalitis of neurologists. Each had their own diseases and their own vocabulary. Now it is only when contemporary photographs of the two conditions are compared (Figure 2)—a patient with schizophrenia (dementia praecox) in a psychiatric textbook (Norman 1928) and a post-encephalitic patient in a contemporary neurology textbook (Wilson 1940)—that the similarities between the two conditions are seen to be much more striking than contemporary written accounts would suggest.

The relationship between encephalitis and schizophrenia was well analysed by Vermeylen in 1938 (Vermeylen 1938). He felt that the viewpoint, psychological or neurological, of different observers influenced their opinion of this relationship. Depending on the conceptual viewpoint of the observer, the neuropsychiatric sequelae of epidemic encephalitis were, for some, kept rigidly separated conceptually from the similar manifestations of schizophrenia and, for others, considered one and the same thing.

Dr Richard Hunter who worked at Friern hospital in North London in the 1960s and 1970s was an interesting psychiatrist. Having started his career with an interest in psychodynamic psychiatry he had, by the end of it, adopted a completely neurological approach for any serious psychiatric disorder. He then never allowed a diagnosis of schizophrenia in any of his patients. Many of his long-stay patients had been patients in the hospital long before he joined the staff, some from the beginning of the century, and most of these had been diagnosed as schizophrenic, once schizoprenia had been adopted in this country. For Richard Hunter, they all had encephalitis. This was not on the basis of diagnostic tests for encephalitis but because this diagnosis was more in keeping with his neurological approach. Following his retirement in the 1980s, the care of his patients passed again to more conventional psychiatric consultants and the same patients received once again conventional psychiatric diagnoses including schizophrenia. So a considerable number of patients received successive diagnoses of schizophrenia, encephalitis and schizophrenia again, depending on who was caring for them.

Hunter did perform extensive investigations on his patients, but this did not help to resolve the issue.

A.B. was first admitted to Friern under Richard Hunter in 1965 at the age of 41. Three months before, he had had a flu-like illness followed by personality change and paranoid delusions, and was admitted after he tried to set fire to himself and his mother. His neurological examination was normal at this stage. Six months after first admission he was treated with chlorpromazine—3 months later he would stand immobile for hours, hunched up and drooling saliva with involuntary movements of the head. He was investigated with a presumptive diagnosis of encephalitis. One of three electro-encephalograms (EEG) showed a non-specific abnormality. One of eight lumbar punctures showed a mild elevation of total protein. Air encephalography showed mild atrophy. A brain biopsy showed mild, non-specific abnormalities. He was seen at the National Hospital, Queen Square, where a diagnosis of sporadic encephalitis lethargica was made and confirmed by neurological colleagues, including Dr Macdonald Critchley who had personal experience of the epidemic cases of encephalitis lethargica in the 1920s. The patient returned to Friern where he did not really stand out from other chronic patients on his ward. After Richard Hunter's death, most of his patients were re-diagnosed as having schizophrenia, including patient A.B.

One of Hunter's wards did retain the designation 'neurological' after he had left. The history of this ward is interesting. Hunter had taken over the care of the ward to which, for a considerable period of time, the most difficult patients in the hospital had been transferred for administrative reasons. The average length of admission of these patients was over 40 years. Now with a considerable number in their sixties and seventies, their defect states were so florid that they acquired a neurological designation from the administration. Examination of the patients and their case notes, however, showed that specific neurological diagnoses could not be made for any of them, that their diagnosis before Hunter took over their care had been schizophrenia, and that their clinical features, including features of possible neurological disorder, differed in degree but not in kind from the rest of the patients with similar lengths of admission to the hospital.

Richard Hunter may simply have been ahead of his time and psychiatry is now catching up with him. In a recent article in the *British Journal of Psychiatry* (Johnson & Lucey 1987) there is a report of two cases of sporadic contemporary encephalitis lethargica. They presented with depressive and catatonic features. The only abnormality on investigation was an abnormal EEG in one case, which improved after a course of electroconvulsive therapy (ECT). The only evidence to support a diagnosis of encephalitis by the authors was their statement that it was now generally accepted that catatonic states are symptomatic of a neurological illness. It was only in 1972 (Arieti 1972) that catatonia was identified as predominantly a disorder of the will and not a disorder of the motor apparatus.

A CONFLICT OF PARADIGMS

Such a conceptual divide is well analysed in Thomas Kuhn's account of conceptual frameworks in science, or 'paradigms', which has won widespread support among historians and philosophers of science (Kuhn 1970). Paradigms are necessary to make most sense of the currently available facts in any particular field of science. They are not facts but ways of making sense of facts. For most of the time researchers in a particular field work within one accepted paradigm. This is what Kuhn calls 'normal science', when conceptual issues in that field are not at issue and workers in the field are happy to extend knowledge within the accepted paradigm.

At certain times in a particular field of science, however, different paradigms are able to make most sense of the same facts and these are then rivals. An example would be when Einstein proposed a new paradigm in the field of physics to replace the previously accepted paradigm of Newton. This leads to a period of conflict between the two paradigms, when different workers work within one or other paradigm. A characteristic of this situation is that workers within different paradigms in the same field cannot talk meaningfully to each other about the same facts. Their vocabulary is not congruent.

This is exactly the state of affairs that has existed in psychiatry over the last 100 years. Rival neurological and psychological explanatory paradigms have been in conflict. A good visual analogy for these rival paradigms is the Necker cube, with its two rival perspectives, shown in Figure 3. The distinction between a neurological or psychological conception of any psychiatric disorder, between the two views of the Necker cube, cannot be resolved by any amount of factual information. The two different perspectives of the Necker cube, just like the two different views of psychiatric disorder, are different ways of making sense of the same facts. The two rival views are equally valid but at the same time they are mutually exclusive. One cannot view both perspectives of the cube, front face bottom left or front face top right, at the same time. Likewise, psychological and neurological paradigms for making sense of psychiatric disorder are equally valid but mutually exclusive.

This conflict between rival neurological and psychological paradigms applies to individual patients with psychiatric disorder, particular psychiatric disorders and psychiatric disorder in general.

> When I started one of my first training posts in psychiatry, the consultant told me that a patient of his on a ward of patients with chronic schizophrenia had previously been investigated and found to have cerebral lupus but it had not been recorded in the notes and he had forgotten which one. All the patients had a diagnosis of schizophrenia again. I had to perform blood tests on all the patients to try and find out which one, in fact, 'really' had lupus.

Here, the Necker cube switched several times in the case of an individual patient.

Majority opinion about whether particular psychiatric disorders or psychiatric disorder generally are best viewed from a neurological or a psychological paradigm is subject to a historical process. The most popular paradigm in terms of majority opinion at any particular time can be called the 'prevalent paradigm'. Between 1890 and 1910, the neurological paradigm of Griesinger and Maudsley was replaced as prevalent paradigm by a psychological paradigm. From the mid 1960s, the process has been reversed.

Conversion from one paradigm to the other, a switch in perspective of the psychiatric Necker cube, is rare but does occur:

> Symptoms which I had looked upon in my patients for many years, and had accepted as the bizarre or stereotyped behaviour of schizophrenics, and which I had conscientiously tried to interpret psychodynamically, now increasingly appeared to me similar, if not actually identical with, known organically determined symptoms (Anderson 1952).

Camilla Anderson was a child psychiatrist. The change in prevalent paradigm for childhood psychosis she is describing, from a psychological to a neurological one, occurred between 1950 and 1970, a generation ahead of the change for adult psychosis. Conflict between two rival paradigms is usually resolved by one replacing the other as prevalent paradigm over the course of a generation, as one generation with a particular paradigm retires and a new generation with a different paradigm takes over. While both paradigms co-exist, there is potential conflict between them which cannot be resolved by any amount of factual information. Even rational discussion is difficult if the presence of irreconcilable paradigms is not recognised. This situation is often met and can result in much non-productive discussion.

Kuhn compares conversions from one paradigm to another to religious conversions. The conflict of paradigms in psychiatry this century has given rise to decidedly 'non-scientific' argument. Karl Kleist, a disciple of Carl Wernicke, carried on the nineteenth century tradition of seeking to apply neurological thinking to psychiatric symptomatology, against the prevailing tide, right up to the time of his death in 1960. Here is a quotation about him from a paper in the 1960s by an eminent neurologist on the neurology of psychotic speech:

> ...at one time some continental neuro-psychiatrists ...were tempted to visualize a linguistic pathophysiology and even a morbid anatomy as an explanation of the aphasia-like states of schizophrenia. Kleist, for example, speculated that there might be cortico-subcortical changes to account for the speech impairment and he even attributed some of the iterative and perseveratory phenomena to lesions within the basal ganglia. These notions never received credence and rightly so: Kleist in his neurological thinking had always been a deviationist, a heretic and a materialist (Critchley 1964).

A psychological paradigm for making most sense in understanding a particular psychiatric disorder should not be confused with psychological precipitants for psychiatric disorder, which are compatible with both psychological and neurological conceptions of psychiatric disorder. Take the following case:

> C.D. was born in Poland in 1913. She saw her parents being killed in an anti-Jewish pogrom when she was 7 years old. She came to England and was adopted at the age of 13 years. She was healthy and did well at school, being noted to have above average intelligence. At the age of 15 years, she was taken to a lecture in Covent

Garden where massacres in Russia were described. Four to five days later, she became depressed, lethargic and then disorientated, with incoherent speech. She was admitted to the National Hospital, Queen Square, where no abnormality was found on investigation. She was admitted to Friern psychiatric hospital 7 weeks after the first symptom had appeared, with a diagnosis of schizophrenia. She stayed there continuously with an unremitting severe schizophrenic illness for over 50 years. She neither spoke nor entered into any conversation, although she rambled incoherently. She had phases of catatonic excitement when her speech was confined to making animal-like noises and she would attack anyone within reach without provocation, kicking, hitting or scratching her victim with the utmost ferocity. At other times she would grunt, lying huddled up in an 'embryo-foetal' position. She was confused and incontinent. Early on, she was deemed to be mentally defective, despite her premorbid history of above average intelligence, and later, profoundly demented. Different physical treatments were tried as they appeared: cardiazol fits, leucotomy, electro-convulsive therapy and neuroleptic medication. Each produced some temporary but never sustained or significant improvement. No neurological features were ever noted except for a single epileptic seizure following her leucotomy.

This schizophrenic disorder clearly seems to have been irreversibly precipitated by psychological trauma. This does not determine whether a psychological or, as is currently increasingly the case, a neurological paradigm is adopted for understanding schizophrenic disorder. Whether a particular disorder is precipitated or relieved by psychological factors has no bearing on whether a neurological or psychological paradigm is more appropriate for understanding it.

The popularity of a psychological approach to psychiatric disorder at the beginning of this century can perhaps in part be seen as a desire for a 'short cut' to understanding of psychiatric disorder, since satisfying explanations in brain terms were not yet available. However, following the 'trailblazers' who explored the new psychological approach in psychiatry with no lack of neurological knowledge, came subsequent generations for whom the psychological approach was their only possible approach. Psychiatry and neurology developed along separate lines with little interaction or cross-fertilisation of ideas between them, to the detriment of both. The investigation and understanding of psychiatric motor disorder became completely divorced from that of motor disorder in neurological illness and interest in the motor disorder of psychiatric illness, which sat rather uncomfortably in a purely psychological approach, generally declined. Since a neurological paradigm in psychiatry is now gaining ground again and we are heading back to the position of Griesinger and Maudsley, this situation needs to be reversed.

2 Catatonia and Extrapyramidal Disorder

CATATONIA

While the cerebral basis of what is now accepted as neurological extrapyramidal motor disorder was being established during the latter part of the nineteenth century, the formulation of what is still accepted as the archetypal psychiatric motor disorder—catatonia—was first put forward by Ludwig Kahlbaum in 1874 (Kahlbaum 1874). For Kahlbaum, catatonia was a neurological disorder accompanied by psychiatric symptoms. Others agreed. Roller, for example, in 1884 suggested that catatonic motor symptoms were the result of subcortical influence on the cortex. Kraepelin, who included catatonia in the group of deteriorating psychoses, which he called 'dementia praecox' (Kraepelin 1919), adopted an ambivalent conceptual position towards this motor disorder.

The renaming of dementia praecox to schizophrenia by Eugen Bleuler in his 1911 monograph (Bleuler 1911) marked a definite change of paradigm for this disorder. Its motor symptoms now became completely dependent on psychic factors for their origin. Schnautzkrampf or protrusion of the lips, for example, was to be understood as an expression of contempt rather than as a localised tonic contraction of the peri-oral muscles. Attempts by others, such as Kleist, to continue to suggest a cerebral basis for them were repudiated. From then on catatonia was regarded as disorder of the will and explained in terms of the operation of unconscious mental forces, and interest in its clinical features languished. The appearance of catatonic symptoms in other disorders, such as confusional states and general paralysis of the insane (neurosyphilis), was treated merely as a curiosity.

The psychological paradigm was adopted most avidly by Anglo-American authors. Jelliffe and White's treatment of schizophrenia in their 1917 textbook of neurology and psychiatry (Jelliffe & White 1917) was typical. They felt that what was necessary to make the apparently bizarre symptoms of dementia praecox understandable was to 'penetrate beneath the surface indications which the patient manifests and find out their true meaning'. Failure of voluntary attention, lack of interest and disturbances of orientation and memory were explained in terms of withdrawal from reality. Increased suggestibility and muscular rigidity were ways of shutting out the world of reality. Stupor, complete cessation of activity, was a still more effective way. A patient who had to be fed by placing

his food before him and a spoon in his hand and repeating each time the
command to take another mouthful did this because it 'permitted him to remain
within himself'. Abnormal movements, mannerisms and stereotypes, were
indicators of subconscious conflict—they all had their psychological meaning:

> . . . an old precox was observed to keep pounding one hand with her clenched fist
> in a rhythmic stereotyped fashion. It was discovered that in her earlier days she had
> been jilted by a shoemaker. This peculiar action could be seen, in the light of this
> knowledge, as but the movements of the shoemaker pounding at his last (Jelliffe &
> White 1917).

In the sixth edition of their textbook published in 1935, although they still felt
that 'the key to the situation lies in the unconscious', following the appreciation
of subcortical disorder, such as Wilson's disease, double athetosis and torsion
spasm, producing psychiatric symptoms, and catatonic symptoms being found in
neurological illnesses involving basal ganglia pathology, such as cerebral anoxia,
carbon monoxide poisoning and encephalitis lethargica, they suggested that
catatonia was not specific to schizophrenia and that basal ganglia disorder could
be involved. This approach, however, never took hold of the general imagination
in the way that the psychological interpretations of the same symptoms had at the
beginning of the century. Jelliffe and White had always accepted that a considerable number of schizophrenic patients showed marked physical symptoms and not
infrequently had all the outward appearances of being quite ill. They described,
for example, catatonic excitement leading to a rapid failure of nutrition, epileptiform seizures and death. Others, however, extended psychological explanations
even to such fatal catatonic disorder:

> Acute exhaustive psychosis (fatal catatonia) is a psychogenic illness originating in a
> need for self-annihilation as a solution to a problem (Adland 1947).

The divide in the middle part of this century between mainland European and
Anglo-American psychiatric investigators was well shown at the First International
Congress of Neuropathology in Rome in 1952 (Proceedings 1952), which devoted
a whole section to the histopathology of schizophrenia. European investigators
maintained, just as they had at the turn of the century, that catatonic schizophrenia was associated with pathological changes in the basal ganglia. American
and British neuropathologists at the congress were sceptical of neuropathological
changes in schizophrenia. European authors such as Kleist continued to insist on
a cerebral basis for schizophrenia, as he had done from the beginning of the
century, and maintained that motor features of schizophrenia were analogous to
the motor disorders of basal ganglia disease (Kleist 1960). This had little impact
on mainstream Anglo-American psychiatry. With the favouring of a psychological
paradigm for explaining psychiatric disorder went a relative lack of clinical interest

in catatonia, and this was especially marked in the Anglo-American literature (Morrison 1973).

In the 1950s a new cause was suggested for the motor disorder of chronic hospitalised patients—the hospital environment itself. Following Martin's 1955 *Lancet* article on institutionalisation came Barton's famous monograph on institutional neurosis (Barton 1976). Barton suggested that prolonged stay in hospital produced a characteristic posture with the hands held across the body, the shoulders drooped and the head held forward. Other features of the syndrome were apathy and lack of initiative, producing in severe cases mutism and stupor, aggressive outbursts and shuffling gait. Barton felt that the term 'institution' should not be restricted to collections of buildings, such as mental hospitals, but embraced 'marriage, religion, benevolence, due process, justice, customs and mores and so forth'. An experimental study by Wing and Brown in 1960, comparing chronic schizophrenic patients in different hospital settings, found a strong association between poverty of social environment and clinical features, such as blunted affect, poverty of speech and social withdrawal. They followed this with a series of further studies and a book called *Institutionalism and Schizophrenia*.

Later experimental studies of institutionalisation did not support such a strong association between the social environment and clinical features of long-stay patients. Johnstone and her colleagues (Johnstone et al. 1981) studied 120 patients with a mean duration of schizophrenic illness of 13.8 years, 5–9 years after discharge from hospital compared to 510 in-patients with equal severity of schizophrenic illness. When factors of age and duration of illness were taken into account, there was no difference between the two groups in terms of positive or negative schizophrenic features or behavioural performance. The authors suggested that the deficits of chronic schizophrenia are an integral feature of the disease process and that any effects of institutionalisation are relatively small. A recent study (Curson et al. 1992) tried to replicate the findings of Wing and Brown in their 1960s studies but was unable to do so. Professor Wing, commenting on this study (Wing 1992), regretted the title *Institutionalism and Schizophrenia*, which they had given their book at the time.

This social explanation of the motor features of psychiatric disorder can be seen as a late development of the psychological paradigm which held sway until the 1960s. The introduction of neuroleptic medication in the 1950s also, paradoxically, helped to support the prevalent psychosocial paradigm. Very soon most patients with psychiatric disorder of any severity had been treated with neuroleptic medication and it was then possible to ascribe any motor disorder in these patients to the medication they were given rather than the psychiatric illness from which they were suffering. Significantly, very little experimental evaluation of the similarities and differences between drug and disease based motor disorder was carried out at a time when untreated control groups would have been much more available.

With the change in prevalent paradigm back to a brain-based one for psychiatry starting in the 1960s, catatonia associated with cerebral disorder became of greater interest. The list of possible physical disorders associated with catatonia is considerable and new associations continue to be reported. The known associations were well reviewed by Gelenberg (Gelenberg 1976). They include neurological disorders involving focal lesions of brain-stem, basal ganglia, thalamus, limbic system, temporal and frontal lobes, due to encephalitis, tumours, haemorrhage and other vascular lesions, and diffuse cerebral disorders due to closed head injury, encephalomalacia, epilepsy and neurosyphilis. They also include systemic disorders including hormonal disorders, vitamin deficiency, porphyria, renal and liver failure, and toxicity due to carbon monoxide poisoning, drugs of abuse and neuroleptic medication. Catatonia associated with these recognised cerebral 'organic' disorders is indistinguishable from that associated with 'functional' disorders, the position that Jelliffe and White had finally arrived at 40 years before.

Catatonia also became generally accepted as forming part of a far wider spectrum of psychiatric disorder than a subtype of schizophrenia. For those who could not 'switch paradigms' to a neurological approach for psychiatric disorder, the presence of catatonia in different psychiatric disorders, once this was accepted as undoubted cerebral disorder, posed a problem for which various solutions were offered. The incidence of catatonic schizophrenia was felt to have declined considerably, and its previous presence in patients with schizophrenia or manic–depressive disorder was explained away by the previous inclusion of patients with organic neurological disease in populations of psychotic patients or the 'fortuitous adding on' of epidemic and endemic encephalitic illnesses (Mahendra 1981).

Evidence about the 'decline' of catatonia is not clear-cut. Kraepelin (Kraepelin 1919) diagnosed catatonic schizophrenia in 19.5% of 500 patients with schizophrenia still hospitalised after 12 months. Achte (Achte 1961) compared 100 randomly selected patients under 35 years of age, who were admitted with a diagnosis of schizophrenia at one hospital in Finland from 1933 to 1935, with 100 patients, similarly selected, admitted to the same hospital from 1953 to 1955: 37% of cases from the 1930s were diagnosed catatonic and 11% from the 1950s. Morrison (Morrison 1974) reviewed the admissions to a general psychiatric hospital in the United States between 1920 and 1966. Comparing the first and second halves of this period, the percentage of schizophrenic patients receiving a subtype diagnosis of catatonia dropped from 14 to 8%. Hogarty and Gross (Hogarty & Gross 1966) compared 140 first-admitted schizophrenic patients in 1953 to 166 first admitted with the same diagnosis to the same hospital in 1960: 38% in 1953 were diagnosed catatonic and 25% in 1960. Guggenheim and Babigian (Guggenheim & Babigian 1974) surveyed the Monroe County Psychiatric Case Register, which has data on almost all residents of a representative area of the United States seen in its various in-patient and out-patient psychiatric facilities since 1960. Over an 18-year span from 1948 to 1966 at the university hospital, there had been no major drop in the number of new catatonic schizophrenia cases seen. The prevalence of catatonic to schizophrenia over the 7-year period from 1960 to 1966 remained at 1 per 1000 county inhabitants. This represented 5% of all first diagnoses of schizophrenia, 10% of all diagnoses of schizophrenia and 16% of all persistently hospitalised patients with schizophrenia over this period. This figure of 16% is not so different to Kraepelin's equivalent figure of 19.5% at the beginning of the century.

These studies, while all showing a decreasing prevalence of catatonic schizophrenia did not suggest that the condition was disappearing and did not rule out the possibility that different prevalences in different populations at different times were simply the reflection of differing severity of schizophrenic illness in these differing populations, and the beneficial effects of neuroleptic medication introduced in the 1950s. Equally, the argument that catatonic phenomena in schizophrenic patients was due to the previous inclusion of patients with organic neurological disease in populations of psychotic patients or the 'fortuitous adding on' of epidemic and endemic encephalitic illnesses does not stand up to close scrutiny.

The problem of distinguishing so-called idiopathic schizophrenia and similar disorder associated with known cerebral disorder was appreciated and discussed in published studies throughout the period under review. The cerebral disorders in question were well known to previous authors and, in the case of neurosyphilis and post-encephalitic parkinsonism, for example, much better known by first-hand experience than to present-day authors. The superposition of encephalitis lethargica on pre-existing schizophrenia was described at the time of the epidemic (Dretler 1935). Rather than the production of new features, however, it resulted in the improvement of certain pre-existing features of the schizophrenic illness. This is an interesting finding in view of the later discovered analogies between the effects of neuroleptic medication and post-encephalitic parkinsonism. The possibility of following up this interesting analogy of action is lost, however, if the effects of superposition of encephalitis lethargica on pre-existing schizophrenia are only invoked to explain away awkward findings of motor disorder in schizophrenic patients, rather than being the subject of study in their own right.

BASAL GANGLIA AND PSYCHIATRIC DISORDER

The term 'basal ganglia' was introduced by Ringer in 1879 to describe the putamen and globus pallidus. Other authors included a number of adjacent structures including caudate nucleus, thalamus, habenular ganglion and the subthalamic nucleus of Luys. The caudate nucleus and putamen together were also known as the striatum and the caudate nucleus, putamen and globus pallidus as the corpus striatum. The first experimental work on the function of the basal ganglia was reported in the 1830s. From this time, basal ganglia lesions were reported in a succession of neurological disorders: pseudobulbar palsy by Bright in 1831, Parkinson's disease by Oppolzer in 1861, chorea by Broadbent in 1865, athetosis by Gowers in 1876 and pseudosclerosis, later to be called Wilson's disease, by Westphal in 1883. The significance of these lesions, however, remained unclear since post-mortem examination of other patients with these conditions showed no gross disorder of the basal ganglia and gross lesions could be found in the basal ganglia of people who had shown no evidence of motor disorder.

Lewy (Lewy 1942) reviewed this early work as an introduction to the 1940 meeting of the Association for Research in Nervous and Mental Disease, which was devoted entirely to diseases of the basal ganglia. He felt that the turning point in understanding the function of the basal ganglia came in 1912 when the journal *Brain* published Kinnier Wilson's MD thesis on progressive lenticular disease, the disease which now bears his name (Wilson 1912). He described this paper as marking the point when the 'gestalt' of the basal ganglia suddenly became apparent, but this gestalt was a neurological one—psychiatry was completely left out of the picture. In his otherwise detailed historical account, Lewy makes no mention of reports such as that of Lehmann on pathological findings in the basal ganglia of patients with catatonic schizophrenia in 1898, contemporary with Oppenheim's descriptions of pathological findings in the basal ganglia with athetosis and chorea. In the whole proceedings of the 1940 meeting there is not a single mention of psychiatric disorder.

In his 1912 paper, Wilson introduced a new concept—extrapyramidal motor disorder. Up till then, neurological 'organic' motor disorder had been limited to paralysis, produced by lesions of the pyramidal tract. Wilson suggested that a much wider spectrum of motor disorder could be produced by cerebral disorder, which he called extrapyramidal motor disorder. This included disorders, which up till this period had been regarded as psychiatric or functional, such as Parkinson's disease as well as his new disease. He suggested that gross anatomical lesions were not necessary to produce extrapyramidal disorder, but that dynamic modification of neuronal function was enough. This was less than a decade after the first suggestion of chemical neurotransmission (Elliot 1904).

Of the 12 patients Wilson described with his new extrapyramidal disease 8 had, in addition to prominent motor disorder, prominent psychiatric symptoms with previous diagnoses such as hysteria and schizophrenia. The first attempt to look specifically at the psychiatric disorder accompanying known basal ganglia diseases had to wait till 1947 when Brenner and his colleagues published their study of 17 patients with Wilson's disease, Huntington's chorea, dystonia musculorum deformans and double athetosis (Brenner et al. 1947). The characteristic feature of these psychiatric accompaniments was their variability. The only consistent feature was the effect of their psychic state on their neurological abnormal movements. The movements were typically more prominent with emotional excitement and less prominent with distraction. The authors pointed out that this feature had, up till then, been a hallmark of psychiatric conditions such as hysteria, but that in fact it was a hallmark of basal ganglia disorder. A corollary of this was that psychological forms of treatment could have a role even in progressive disease of the central nervous system; it was the rigid division of psychiatric and neurological disorder that had restricted interest in the role of psychological factors in aggravating or alleviating neurological disorder.

The 1960s saw major advances in the understanding of the anatomy and neurochemistry of the basal ganglia. Anatomical studies showed a highly organised neuronal projection to the basal ganglia from all areas of cortex. Projection from neocortex suggested a cognitive input to motor function, and projection from limbic cortex an affective input. The basal ganglia were shown to contain by far the highest concentration of dopamine in the brain, and ascending projection systems from brain stem to basal ganglia to have dopamine as their major neurotransmitter. These projection systems consisted of the nigrostriatal tract, projecting to the striatum, and the mesolimbic system. The mesolimbic system projected to the anterior extremity of the basal ganglia or limbic striatum, consisting of nucleus accumbens, olfactory tubercle and nucleus of the stria terminalis. These structures were then added to the constituents of the basal ganglia. They also received inputs from the limbic cortex, amygdala and hippocampus.

At the same time, new ideas were put forward for the function of the basal ganglia. The importance of the basal ganglia in processing sensory input as well as motor function had become evident. The description and concept of the reticular activating system put forward by Moruzzi and Magoun in 1949 had revolutionised concepts of vigilance and consciousness. It became accepted that, under normal conscious conditions, each cortical region receives two sets of impulses during the processes of perception, conception and intentional motor action. One set comes through the specific thalamo-cortical projection of the different sensory or other integrative pathways, and one through the non-specific trunco-thalamic projections which travel through the basal ganglia and determine the degree of vigilance and awareness. Only if both sets of impulses arrive at a distinct cortical region, is conscious perception or realisation possible. The basal ganglia control intentional action and not simple movements without conscious representation. They allow attention to be focused on single events with their emotional concomitants by suppressing other happenings and their emotional significance.

With the change to a more brain-based approach to psychiatric disorder, interest in the possible contribution of basal ganglia dysfunction to psychiatric disorder began to grow again. The proceedings of the second meeting of the Association for Research in Nervous and Mental Diseases devoted entirely to the basal ganglia in 1976 (Yahr 1976) contained three paragraphs of discussion on the psychiatric consequences of basal ganglia disease. Histological changes in the basal ganglia of patients with schizophrenia, especially with catatonic features, began to reappear (Stevens 1982). Explanations of psychiatric symptoms in terms of breakdown of basal ganglia function, such as gating sensory input to affect motor behaviour, were suggested (Schneider 1984). Basal ganglia disorder became implicated in other psychiatric disorders, such as obsessive–compulsive disorder, affective disorder, and personality and behaviour disorder. Laplane and his colleagues, in a recent article in *Brain* (Laplane et al. 1989), suggested, like their predecessors in the 1920s, that basal ganglia lesions can give rise to a clinical picture that can be purely motor, purely behavioural or both and that aspects of psychiatric disorders, such as severe depression, catatonic schizophrenia and obsessive–compulsive disorder, could be related to structural and physiological disturbances in the systems linking the frontal associative cortex and the basal ganglia.

It is becoming clear that there is no one characteristic psychiatric disorder associated with the basal ganglia (Rogers 1990). Basal ganglia diseases are associated with a wide variety of psychiatric disorder and basal ganglia disorder contributes to a wide spectrum of psychiatric diseases. Psychiatry is at present in the same position *vis-à-vis* the basal ganglia that neurology found itself in at the end of the last century, from the point of view of movement disorders. There is strong circumstantial evidence linking the two but no definite and invariable association between particular basal ganglia disorder and particular psychiatric disorder. Kinnier Wilson, in 1925 (Wilson 1925), pointed out that lesions of the corpus striatum did not produce any clear-cut symptomatology. Its vascular supply was not derived from a single source, and morbid processes involving its cell and fibre systems were not restricted to the basal ganglia. Now that we are in the neurotransmitter era with emphasis on topographically diffuse, neurotransmitter-based neuronal systems, rather than topographically discrete anatomical systems, it is easier to understand how pathological insults to the basal ganglia can produce variable disruption of different neurotransmitter systems involving the basal ganglia and, therefore, variable clinical effects.

DYSTONIA

One extrapyramidal disorder that has only recently crossed the neurological rubicon is dystonia, which is an excellent example of the Necker cube phenomenon. It was regarded for most of this century from a psychological paradigm—patients with blepharospasm, or screwing up of the eyes, could not look at reality; those with torticollis, or deviation of the head, could not face the future. A neurological paradigm is now favoured, though no convincing pathological change has yet been identified or biochemical basis established, leaving the entire concept of dystonia as one based on clinical evaluation (Marsden 1976). Dystonic disorder can be precipitated, exacerbated, improved or completely resolved by psychosocial factors.

> E.F., a 17 year-old girl who had always held her pen awkwardly when she wrote, developed abnormal hyperpronation movements of one arm when she walked with her boyfriend. These were interpreted as symbolic of an unconscious rejection of him. A few months later she was having a violent argument with the same boyfriend, flung her engagement ring to the ground and turned to walk away from him and, from that moment, was permanently afflicted with a generalised torsion dystonia. She could walk backwards normally but not forwards.

Oculogyric crises, dystonic conjugate spasms of the eyes, were often 'contagious' in a ward with post-encephalitics. When one patient would go into crisis it could set off other patients on the same ward, even when they had never suffered them before. The crises could also be triggered by the sight of certain people, hypnotism or emotional trauma and resolved by simple suggestion or injections of distilled water (Delbeke & Bogaert 1928).

G.H. developed writer's cramp between the ages of 10 and 13, after two forearm fractures of her dominant arm and during a period that she was being sexually abused by her father. The writer's cramp then disappeared but reappeared when she was 35, when her father's impending death from an incurable lymphoma created ambivalent feelings of grief and hatred towards him because of the previous abuse. The writer's cramp persisted after her father's death for 3 years until, with counselling about her feelings towards her father over a period of 12 months, it completely resolved.

A stoical and 'singularly un-neurotic' 46-year-old former pilot with a history of neck injuries developed spasmodic torticollis at the age of 21. His condition slowly deteriorated over the next 10 years. Many different medications were unsuccessful. At the age of 38, after a mass healing service in Los Angeles there was a sudden improvement. Complete resolution occurred over the next 10 days and this was maintained for at least 7 years (Jayne et al. 1984).

In recent double-blind trials of botulinum toxin for spasmodic torticollis, patients are described who improve with placebo injections, including one patient who showed a marked and lasting improvement of his torticollis after the second placebo injection (Jankovic & Orman 1987).

Stanley Fahn, who with David Marsden has done much to win acceptance of dystonia as a neurological disorder, describes torsion dystonia as being mistaken for a conversion disorder probably more often than any other neurological condition, with different surveys indicating that approximately 40% of all patients with this disorder have been so 'misdiagnosed' (Fahn et al. 1983). However, he puts forward 'hysterical dystonia' as a separate 'true conversion disorder', on the grounds of relief of the symptoms by psychotherapy or by supportive and suggestive therapy. This is logically indefensible. Any dystonic disorder could legitimately be regarded as either neurological or psychological, depending on the point of view or paradigm of the observer. No criteria can determine one view as more correct than the other. The absence of recognisable cerebral pathology on investigation or post-mortem examination is no bar to viewing dystonia as a neurological disorder, and nor should it be for psychiatric disorder.

CATATONIA—AN EXTRAPYRAMIDAL DISORDER

For a short period after the appearance of epidemic encephalitis, the similarity between its motor sequelae and the catatonic syndrome struck several observers and there was a flowering of a neurological approach to catatonia. This lasted into the 1930s but then faded as the soil in contemporary psychiatry was not propitious.

Dide and his French colleagues published one of the first of these studies (Dide et al. 1921). They described 12 patients with catatonic schizophrenia whose motor disorder showed interesting analogies with Parkinson's disease. They rejected psychological interpretations of these phenomena, preferring an explanation in terms of cerebral pathology in the basal ganglia and sub-optic areas and maintained that their neuropathological investigations of schizophrenic patients had invariably shown pathology of these cerebral areas more marked than any associated cortical disturbance.

Paul Guiraud (Guiraud 1924), one of these authors, felt that the frequent appearance of catatonic symptoms in epidemic encephalitis, as well as the study of basal ganglia disorder in other conditions such as Wilson's disease, made renewed interest in the neurological basis of catatonia, as favoured by its original proponents, timely. He suggested that the catatonic syndrome should take its place as an extrapyramidal disorder alongside chorea and athetotic syndromes, Wilson's disease and the extrapyramidal disorder with the closest analogies with catatonia, post-encephalitic parkinsonism. Guiraud included the following features in the catatonic syndrome:

- Increased tone.
- Persistence of passively or actively induced postures.
- Arrest of movement.
- Negativism.
- Overcompliance.
- Motor perseveration and stereotypies.
- Mannerisms.
- Echolalia and echopraxia.
- Disorder of facial expression.
- Vasomotor and trophic disorders.

He felt that all these features could be explained by the cardinal features which had been established for extrapyramidal disorder resulting from basal ganglia pathology:

- Loss of harmony of complex movements.
- Increased tone.
- Disorder of facial expression.
- Abnormal involuntary movements.
- Involuntary acceleration and repetition of movements.
- Vasomotor and trophic disorder.

He felt that psychological and neurological ways of seeing catatonic symptoms were radically distinct. The main reason for the currently favoured psychological approach was because catatonia was often associated with obvious mental disorder, whereas in accepted extrapyramidal disorder the psychiatric associations were less marked. However, instead of this 'retreat into the psychological', he favoured attempting to use the association of motor and mental disorder in catatonia to determine the contribution of the basal ganglia to psychiatric disorder.

Haskovec, in Prague in 1925 (Haskovec 1925), felt that the motor disorder of catatonia in psychotic illnesses was proof positive of the involvement of basal ganglia pathology. Farran-Ridge, a British psychiatrist in 1926 (Farran-Ridge 1926), drew specific analogies between symptoms in schizophrenia and encephalitis lethargica. He described persistent chewing movements, choreiform movements and abrupt spontaneous movements as common in schizophrenia and rapid fluttering of the upper eyelids and strong, upward, conjugate deviation of the eyeballs, similar to the oculogyric crises described in post-encephalitic parkinsonism, as occurring in some cases. He ascribed these symptoms to pathology of the basal ganglia.

Reiter, in Denmark in 1926 (Reiter 1926), regretted the increasing division between neurology and psychiatry at the time. He felt that the only secure advances in psychiatry, at least for severe psychiatric disorders, such as schizophrenia, were to be made with a neurological approach. The recent epidemic encephalitis he felt had shown that the probable cerebral seat for higher psychical functions was not the cortex, as previously thought, but rather the central grey matter of the brain. The absence of obvious pathological change in this area of the brain in schizophrenia might be, he suggested, because these pathological changes were more chemical than morphological. An overlap between the motor disorder of schizophrenia and encephalitis should be expected and he described prominent extrapyramidal motor disturbances in 10 cases of schizophrenia: in four parkinsonism developed in the early phase of their psychosis and in six, motor disturbances—myoclonus, choreo-athetotic restlessness, tremor, increased tone, hyperreflexia, epileptiform convulsions, contractures and extensor plantar responses—associated with an unknown toxic condition, preceded death by up to a year.

Also in 1926, Hans Steck, in Switzerland (Steck 1926, 1927) published an extensive study of extrapyramidal syndromes in psychiatric illnesses, still the best available assessment of pre-neuroleptic psychiatric motor disorders. These motor syndromes consisted of the variable expression of the following motor abnormalities:

- Akinesia, including immobility, aspontaneity, slowness in the initiation and execution of voluntary movements and decreased responsiveness.
- Hyperkinesia, including increased activity, outbursts, negativism, stereotypies, choreic and athetotic movements.
- Disorder of posture, including flexion, especially of the head, persistence of postures (catalepsy) and contractures of the hands.
- Disorder of tone, including rigidity, waxy flexibility and hypotonias.

- Disorder of facial expression including amimetic facies and frontalis spasm.
- Disorders of speech, including dysarthria, unintelligible speech, mutism, perseveration, palilalia and echolalia.
- Vasomotor disturbance, including oedema and cyanosis.
- Secretomotor disturbance, including seborrhoea, sweating and salivation.
- Pupillary disturbance, including anisocoria, dilatation and impaired reflexes.

These abnormalities were found in a variety of organic syndromes including general paralysis, dementing illnesses and mental subnormality, as well as patients with schizophrenic disorders, where they formed the catatonic syndrome, and other psychiatric disorders, including manic-depressive psychosis, involutional melancholia and hysteria.

Steck characterised these motor syndromes as disorder of the extrapyramidal system comparable to the motor syndromes of Wilson's disease and encephalitis lethargica. He felt that an extrapyramidal motor syndrome formed part of nearly all severe psychiatric illnesses. He saw striking resemblances between epidemic encephalitis, general paralysis of the insane and catatonic schizophrenia, both in their acute excitatory phases and chronic defect states. Disturbance of an identical cerebral system explained why analogous symptoms appeared in conditions of very different aetiology.

In terms of motor disorder, he saw no absolute distinction between catatonic schizophrenia and post-encephalitic parkinsonism. The associated psychiatric disorder of post-encephalitic parkinsonism, however, of which he had also made an extensive study (Steck 1931), was but a rough sketch of that of schizophrenia. Steck accepted the value of psychological insights but insisted on the validity of a neurological approach granted that schizophrenia was a neurological disorder. He eschewed any attempt at precise anatomical cerebral localisation, but suggested that in schizophrenia there was a more widespread cerebral disturbance than in post-encephalitic parkinsonism, with both cortical and sub-cortical involvement. Proof of this hypothesis needed neuropathological demonstration. Lesions in general paralysis of the insane and encephalitis lethargica were pathognomonic, but neuropathological changes in schizophrenia were slight and difficult to interpret. Together with the clinical findings, however, they supported an extrapyramidal basis for the motor disorder of psychiatric illness.

Claude and his colleagues in France (Claude et al. 1927b), after careful experimental work involving the electric excitability of muscles, postural and other reflexes, and pharmacological intervention, felt that the catatonic motor disorder of schizophrenia, although resembling extrapyramidal disorder in various respects, could be clearly distinguished from 'organic' extrapyramidal disorder. It was variable in expression, subject to some voluntary control, and transient. Interestingly, in two of the 25 schizophrenic patients they examined, they found extensor plantar responses, which could likewise be variable in expression, being of sudden onset, coinciding with an exacerbation of the psychotic disorder, and transient, lasting up to several months but then disappearing.

The main distinguishing feature between catatonia and parkinsonism for Claude and his colleagues was that where the parkinsonian patient tried to overcome his disabilities, the catatonic patient did not. They quoted the catatonic patient in remission who when asked why he had not moved during his catatonic period replied that it was because he had not wanted to—he had lost the idea of movement. They suggested that cerebral involvement in catatonia was more widespread than purely basal ganglia, also involving the cortex, and that this involvement was due to dynamic alterations of different cerebral systems, rather than fixed localised disorder which typified accepted neurological disorder.

Others agreed that the mechanism producing catatonia in patients with schizophrenia must be the same as that producing identical symptoms in post-encephalitic parkinsonism. Paradoxical kinesia and catatonic excitement, for example, had to be regarded neurologically as the same (Miller 1927). When it came to 'unconscious volition':

> Forces outside the field of awareness must be regarded as neurological, and such activities, though they may be interpreted as symbolically infantile, are essentially due to the activity of the grey matter of the mid-brain which is no longer under cortical inhibition (Miller 1927).

At the 1928 Congress of Psychiatrists and Neurologists at Anvers in Belgium, Divry (Divry 1928) highlighted the conflict of paradigms regarding the interpretation of catatonic motor disorder:

> The study of catatonia in the light of extrapyramidal disorder brings to the fore a conflict in the interpretation of the catatonic syndrome which first appeared at the end of the last century. Where some see in this motor disorder only the corollary of psychic processes, others suggest a diametrically opposite interpretation which in its most radical form equates the catatonic syndrome with extrapyramidal disorder— subcortical disorder which is not secondary to psychic disorder but on the contrary contributes to psychiatric disorder (Divry 1928).

At the annual meeting of the American Neurological Association in 1929, Samuel Orton argued for a neurological approach to catatonia (Orton 1930). Adolf Meyer, the most influential contemporary American psychiatrist, was a discussant of what he called these 'organicist's musings'. He felt that one of the saddest things to have happened to Kahlbaum was to take general paralysis of the insane as a model for his concept of catatonia. Meyer suggested that a neurological approach should be restricted to defining localised anatomical disorder. The neurologist Foster-Kennedy, also a discussant, defended Orton. He questioned the term 'organicist'. Was it possible, he asked, to differentiate neurologists and psychiatrists so completely? He suggested that neurologists were in fact psychiatrists with insight into their own ignorance. It was presumptuous to assume that because 50 years of histological examination of the brain in psychiatric disorder had not shown any changes, there were, therefore, no structural brain changes.

Some, such as Harriet Babcock (Babcock 1933) were forthright in their criticisms of psychological explanations of psychiatric disorder, calling them inadequate and absurd. Discussing the abnormalities of posture in catatonia, for example, she pointed out that one could withdraw from the world as successfully 'in a comfortable position as in a strained one'. Even Eugen Bleuler had second thoughts. In a lecture delivered in the United States (Bleuler 1930), he said:

> Since Jung and myself, following in Freud's footsteps, pointed out that a great part of the symptomatology of schizophrenia is to be regarded as psychic reaction . . . some of us often inclined to overlook that these psychic mechanisms . . . do not explain the whole disease . . . there are even symptoms that seem to indicate that there must be physiological lesions . . . which are likewise found in various diseases of the basal ganglia (Bleuler 1930).

The remarkable thing from a historical point of view is that neither this 'recantation', nor any of the other studies described, had much if any effect on contemporary psychiatric thought. The psychological paradigm was too entrenched and remained the prevalent one till the mid 1960s.

Exceptions continued to the preoccupation with psychological conceptions of psychiatric disorder. The metabolic changes in cases of periodic catatonia were meticulously investigated by Rolv Gjessing in Norway (Gjessing 1976). Fred Mettler in the United States was ahead of his time in the 1950s, suggesting that the basal ganglia had more a sensori-motor role rather than a purely motor function. He suggested that the schizophrenic syndrome was basically a perceptual disorder caused by dysfunction of the basal ganglia producing secondary cortical dysfunction (Mettler 1955). A full appreciation of neurotransmitter function was still to come, however, and when it came to a possible mechanism to explain the characteristic variability and reversibility of psychiatric symptoms and their relationship with emotional triggers, he could only suggest vasospasm in the basal ganglia.

The 1960s saw the neurotransmitter revolution and a 'scientific revolution' in psychiatry. The relationship between the extrapyramidal system and schizophrenia was taken up again (Kline & Mettler 1961). Klawans and his colleagues (Klawans et al. 1972) suggested that the dopaminergic system in the basal ganglia could be a final common pathway for the schizophrenic syndrome and there should be a relationship between this syndrome and known basal ganglia disorder involving dopaminergic mechanisms. Stevens (Stevens 1973) suggested that schizophrenia could include dysfunction of the mesolimbic dopamine projection system in a manner similar to dysfunction of the nigrostriatal dopamine system in known basal ganglia disorders such as Parkinson's disease. Webster (Webster 1975), at a meeting of the psychiatry section of the Royal Society of Medicine, organised by Richard Hunter and devoted to the basal ganglia, suggested that distinguishing motor activity and behaviour was more a reflection of the particular orientation of different investigators than a meaningful separation of categories in cerebral terms.

Some continued to insist on a sharp division between psychiatric motor disorder and neurological extrapyramidal disorder. Professor David Marsden and his colleagues, in their influential review of spontaneous and drug-induced movement disorders in psychotic patients in 1975 (Marsden et al. 1975), for example, went out of their way to emphasise the distinction between spontaneous and drug-induced motor disorder in these patients. Many of their statements, however, argued against this:

> In certain cases motor disturbances associated with psychosis bear a strong resemblance to abnormal movements appearing in neurological disturbances of the extrapyramidal system . . .

> A superficial resemblance of these stereotypies to oral–facial dyskinesias and choreiform activity of neurologic disorders is frequently apparent . . .

> The akinetic features of catatonic schizophrenia often closely resemble akinetic disorders of the extrapyramidal system . . .

> . . . psychiatry and neurology have an increasing area of common interest, notably including the topics that we have discussed (Marsden et al. 1975)

Arguments for the distinction of motor disorder in psychiatry from neurological disorder required special pleading:

> Such motor activity is obviously more complex and purposeful in appearance than the hyperkinetic dyskinesia occurring in neurological disorders . . .

> . . . the vast majority are best regarded as tic-like disturbances whose repetitive, stereotyped quality differentiates them from chorea, athetosis or dystonia.

> The similarities that have been emphasised, however, appear to be limited to external appearances.

> . . . superficial similarity of appearance does not necessarily indicate a common etiology or pathophysiology for movement disorders in psychiatric and neurological syndromes (Marsden et al. 1975).

Whatever the practical merits of emphasising the differences rather than the similarities between neurological and psychiatric motor disorders, this has had the effect of holding back a much needed neurological approach to the motor disorder of psychiatric illness. By far the best way forward is accepting catatonic motor disorder, whether forming part of neurological or psychiatric disorder, as an extrapyramidal motor disorder (Rogers 1991).

3 Schizophrenia

KAHLBAUM

Our present concept of schizophrenia was shaped by three nearly exact, contemporaries, Emil Kraepelin (1855–1926), Eugen Bleuler (1857–1939) and Sigmund Freud (1856–1939). Their contribution carried on the work of previous psychiatrists, the most significant of whom was Karl Kahlbaum (1828–1899), who was the first to describe hebephrenia in 1863 (followed by further descriptions by his pupil Hecker in 1871), the first to describe catatonia (in lectures at the University of Koenigsberg, in 1866) and who coined the term 'paraphrenia'. Over the second half of the nineteenth century, the concept of dementia praecox, a term first used by Morel in 1860, gradually matured in the work of Kraepelin who, by 1899, had defined it as a distinct disease incorporating hebephrenia, catatonia and paranoia. Our present concept of schizophrenia was finally crystallised by Bleuler, when he set out to apply Freud's ideas to Kraepelin's concept of dementia praecox, renaming it 'schizophrenia' in 1911.

Motor disorder was thus an integral part of schizophrenia from the outset. It was named catatonia by Kahlbaum in his classic monograph *Die Katatonie oder das Spannungsirresein* published in 1874. An English translation only appeared in 1973 (Kahlbaum 1874).

In his monograph, Kahlbaum mentions that he had observed at least 50 cases. The features of 25 cases are given: these are numbered cases 1–14 and 16–26 (where is no case 15). Cases 22–25 are cases of general paralysis with no features of catatonia. A breakdown of motor disorder in the 21 patients described with catatonia is given in Table 3.1.

The motor disorder described by Kahlbaum as 'catatonia' thus included: abnormal postures, typically flexion of the head, and persistence of postures; rigidity and resistance to passive movements; decreased spontaneous activity, motionlessness and decreased responsiveness; general overactivity, outbursts of activity and abnormal activity, such as destructiveness; abnormal movements of trunk and limbs, and of the face, including jerking, twitching, spasms and cramps; abnormal eye movements and gait; abnormal speech production with mutism, decreased spontaneous speech, increased speech production and unintelligible speech.

Table 3.1 Breakdown of motor disorder in 21 patients described with catatonia (after Kahlbaum 1973)

Disorder	Symptom	Case no.
Disorder of posture (17 patients)	Flexion of head	1,6,7,8,17,18,26
	Flexion of trunk	1,3,4,7,13
	Flexion of limbs	3,6,7
	Persistence of postures	1,2,11,14,18,21,26
	Peculiar postures	5,6,11,13,19
	Extension postures	1,16
Disorder of tone (9 patients)	Rigidity, stiffness	1,4,6,12
	Resistance to passive movement	1,2,3,14,17,18
Disorder of motor performance (18 patients)	Decreased activity	1,2,3,4,6,7,8,9,11 14,16,17,18, 19,20,26
	Motionlessness	1,3,4,7,8,9,11,14, 16,17,18,19,26
	Decreased responsiveness	1,2,4,8,10,18,19, 26
	Difficulty initiating	1,5,6,7
Disorder of activity (13 patients)	General overactivity	1,7,13,14,16,20,21
	Outbursts	1,3,4,5,6,11,16
	Destructiveness, self-mutilation, stripping	3,4,5,11,12,16
Abnormal movements of trunk and limbs (10 patients)	Jerking, tics, choreiform twitching	1,2,14,20
	Spasms, cramps	1,2,3,4,11,18
	Seizures, convulsive-like disorder	2,3,4,5,11,19
	Stereotyped activity, gyration	3,11,20
	Tremors	11,14
Abnormal facial movements (11 patients)	Choreiform, twitching, peculiar	1,2,6,26
	Spasms, cramps, contorted	1,2,3,4,5,6,10,14, 26
	Expressionless, flaccid	1,7,8,10
	Fixed expression	1,2,7,14
Abnormal eye movements (7 patients)	Cramps	10
	Rolling, searching	10,16
	Fixed gaze	1,7,8,10,13,26
Abnormal gait (5 patients)	Halting, slow, stiff	1,2,5,6,12
Abnormal speech production (20 patients)	Mutism	1,2,4,6,8,10,12, 14,16,19,26
	Decreased speech	1,3,7,8,9,10,12, 13,14,16,17,18
	Slow speech, delay	1,7
	Increased speech	2,3,4,11,12,21
	Outbursts, swearing	2,6,9,26
	Abnormal volume, timbre	24,7,11,13,20,26
	Unintelligible, sounds, lip movements	3,7,12,13,14

KRAEPELIN

Kahlbaum's catatonia formed one of the three main clinical forms of Kraepelin's dementia praecox. It could not, however, be sharply separated from the remaining forms of dementia praecox because individual catatonic symptoms were often found in other forms of the disease. Catatonic symptoms were also found in many other quite different illnesses, and so were not pathognomonic for dementia praecox. What Kraepelin felt was the hallmark of the catatonic form of dementia praecox was when states of catatonic stupor and excitement dominated the clinical picture. These states of stupor or excitement varied markedly in duration lasting for hours, days, weeks, months or years at a time, and frequency. They could be separated by remission from illness, sometimes lasting for many years, or a defect state, which he called dementia. Thus defined, the catatonic form of dementia praecox formed some 20% of all Kraepelin's cases.

The English translation of Kraepelin's account of dementia praecox first appeared in 1919 (Kraepelin 1919). In this work, Kraepelin divided the symptoms of dementia praecox into psychic and bodily symptoms. Under 'bodily symptoms' were included headaches, pupillary disturbances, tendon reflex changes, aphasia, seizures, spasmodic phenomena, vasomotor disorders, changes in blood pressure, respiration, secretion of saliva, temperature, menstruation, blood, metabolism, sleep and appetite. Also considered were the 'cerebellar' form of dementia praecox and experiments on catalepsy and voluntary finger movements.

Under 'psychic symptoms', he included a weakening of the domain of the will. This produced a variety of different manifestations:

- A loss of independent impulses for work and action, although the capability of action, if stimulated from outside, could be preserved.
- Automatic obedience, when the influence of outside stimulation was marked, including waxy flexibility, the persistence of passively induced postures, and echolalia and echopraxia, the involuntary repetition of words and actions.
- Impulsive actions, which could be sudden and violent.
- Catatonic excitement, persistent 'discharges of will-power', manifested as impulsive actions and aimless, energetic 'mutilated movements of purpose or expression'.
- Stereotypy, or persistence of spontaneous purposeless movements, actions or postures in the absence of normal purposeful movement, including twitching movements of muscles, 'contortionist movements', rhythmic movements such as rocking from one leg to the other and standing or lying in the same position for hours or days.
- Mannerisms or distortion of normal movement including expending too much force or producing clumsy, jerky, stiff, wooden or angular simple movements, or using unnecessary groups of muscles for a movement or unnecessary movements for an action, the aim of the action being wholly or at least partially

frustrated by these abnormalities, so that the action became unrecognisable, odd and apparently senseless.

- Parabulia or derailment of volition, actions not starting, once started stopping before completion, or turning into another action, including those exactly contrary to the action intended or requested.
- A decrease in spontaneous speech, mutism, echolalia, outbursts including swearing and screaming, increased flow and incoherence of speech, stereotypy, with repetition of sentences, words and sounds, clicking, lip smacking, sniffing and snorting, disturbance of flow, modulation or timbre, mutilation of individual words or the construction of sentences so that speech became incomprehensible and negativism including evasive answers such as 'I don't know' to every question, 'speaking past the subject', not being able to start talking in conversation, stopping before completion of an answer and low volume, unintelligible speech.

Thus most of the symptomatology of dementia praecox, including the majority of its motor disorders, were considered by Kraepelin as psychological rather than physical disorders, disorders of the will rather than disorders of the brain. The physical disorders were in the minority and difficult to incorporate with his predominantly psychological conception of the illness. He described spasmodic phenomena of the muscles of the face and speech as extremely peculiar. Grimacing facial movements reminded him of the corresponding disorders of choreic patients. Tremor of the muscles of the mouth could completely resemble that of paralytics. When he considered experiments on persistence of posture under 'bodily symptoms', he had to add the rider that the principal cause of this power of endurance was disorder of volitional impulse. When he described consciousness as clouded in catatonic states, he stressed that these were produced by disorder of volition.

Despite this emphasis on a psychological frame of reference, Kraepelin deals quite extensively with the possible cerebral basis for the condition. He devotes a whole chapter to the morbid anatomy of the condition. In keeping with nineteenth-century views of the cerebral localisation of psychic disorder, he confines his attention to the cortex, concluding that the frontal and temporal cortex bore the brunt of the disease process. The knowledge for any more elaborate neurological explanation was not yet available. Kraepelin, therefore, accepted an ambivalent conceptual position. He was happy to deal with dementia praecox from both a psychological and neurological paradigm. However, he had no time for the contemporary . . .

. . . Freudian trend of investigation, the representation of arbitrary assumptions and conjectures as assured facts, which are used without hesitation for the building up of always new castles in the air ever towering higher, and the tendency to generalisation beyond measure from single observations (Kraepelin 1919).

BLEULER

This was in marked contrast to their contemporary, Bleuler. Bleuler's monograph replacing the term 'dementia praecox' with 'schizophrenia' appeared in 1911 (Bleuler 1911). Straightaway on the first page of his monograph, Bleuler makes clear that an important aspect of his reformulation of Kraepelin's concept was . . .

> . . . nothing less than the application of Freud's ideas to dementia praecox (Bleuler 1911).

Schnautzkrampf, spasm of peri-oral muscles, for example, was an expression of both contempt for the environment and marked self-satisfaction, rather than a localised tonic contraction of the peri-oral muscles. Head movements were displaced coitus movements. The tiny pieces of cloth sewn by a paranoid patient were her thoughts. Kissing other people's shoes or the ground was due to an inferiority complex. Rocking an object held in the arms or simply rocking was connected with a child complex. The frequent episodes of laughing and crying, which Kahlbaum had described as physical symptoms, were an expression of unconsciously operating complexes. Bleuler felt that none of these interpretations was arbitrary and that the validity of interpreting schizophrenic symptoms in terms of Freudian symbolism could be proved 'with the accuracy of an experiment in physics'.

Bleuler's account of schizophrenia first appeared in English in 1923 in the translation by Brill of the fourth edition of his textbook of psychiatry (Bleuler 1923). According to Brill, at Burgholzi where Bleuler worked, psycho-analytic methods were applied to all accessible patients and investigated even in the organic psychoses. The espousal of a completely psychological paradigm led to contradictions and any symptoms suggesting obvious cerebral impairment had to be played down. In schizophrenia, in contrast to the organic psychoses, sensation, memory, consciousness and motility were not directly disturbed, except in very far advanced cases or in an accessory way.

However Bleuler, like Kraepelin, vacillated in his conceptual position. At one point, in his 1911 monograph, he writes that the somatic symptoms found in the disorder suggest that the disease is based upon a fundamental alteration of the brain. Elsewhere in the same monograph he suggests it is not absolutely necessary to assume the presence of a physical disease process since the entire symptomatology could be psychically determined. He discusses the possibility of psychic functions being based on sub-cortical cerebral mechanisms, but only to dismiss it.

Motor disorder was characteristic of patients with schizophrenia. Bleuler could make this diagnosis simply by seeing patients up to the knee behind a hedge because of their gait. He could not, however, go along with the views of those, such as the Wernicke school, who postulated disturbances of motility 'in the strict sense' in schizophrenia, or those, such as Schuele, who located their origin in the deeper parts of the central nervous system. Grimaces of all kinds, peculiar ways of shrugging the shoulder, extraordinary movements of tongue and lips, finger play, sudden involuntary gestures were the reason why some authors had spoken of choreic or tetanic movements in catatonia, 'quite mistakenly, though'. Many of these abnormal movements could not be distinguished from tics, but choreic, athetotic and tetanic phenomena were entirely different from the motor symptoms which accompanied schizophrenia. He had never seen choreal disturbances that belonged to schizophrenia.

How was it, he asked, that individuals who could not even sit up were capable of carrying out complicated, powerful, and correctly co-ordinated locomotion upon some psychic stimulus? Difficulty with purposive movement, as when, instead of combing her hair, a patient ran the comb over her coat, could externally resemble apraxia, but even apraxic symptoms could, he argued, be an expression of a general psychic disturbance. There was no doubt that catalepsy was precipitated by psychic factors. Only such a concept could explain the rapid changes that occurred under psychic influences.

The only two purely motor symptoms he accepted were spasms and idiomuscular contractions. Idio-muscular contraction referred to obvious contraction of muscle bundles, for example, in pectoralis major on light percussion of the muscle. It had been found in up to 95% of patients with dementia praecox. It was also found in 90% of patients with general paralysis, in 12% of patients with manic–depressive psychosis, as well as in normal subjects. There was no known associated pathology and examination of the spinal cord had invariably been normal. It was commoner in men than women. Some maintained that it was associated with dehydration or severe nutritional disturbance. It has not been the subject of much subsequent interest.

Bleuler continued to use Kahlbaum's term 'catatonia' to describe peculiar forms of motility, stupor, mutism, stereotypy, mannerism, negativism, command automatism, spontaneous automatism and impulsivity. He felt that more than half of his institutionalised schizophrenic patients showed catatonic symptoms either transiently or permanently, and he felt that they probably represented increased severity of the disease rather than a distinct syndrome.

LATER AUTHORS

The descriptions by Kahlbaum, Kraepelin and Bleuler became the standard account of catatonic motor disorder in schizophrenia. Jelliffe and White, for example, in their *Textbook of Neurology and Psychiatry* (Jelliffe & White 1917), described catatonia as the variety of dementia praecox with a predominance of motility disturbance, typically an alternation between catatonic stupor and catatonic excitement.

In catatonic stupor the patients could be perfectly immobile, sitting in corners by themselves or lying in bed without paying any apparent attention to what was going on around them, failing to answer questions and not reacting at all to external stimuli. Bladder and rectum would become overloaded and saliva accumulate in the mouth. Abnormal postures were characteristic, called 'attitudinising', with grimacing. Speech when present was incoherent and perseverative. The limbs could stay indefinitely in whatever position they were placed—waxy flexibility or catalepsy. This could be associated with suggestibility and command automatism, automatic and mechanical compliance with any request, echolalia, repetition of words heard, and echopraxia, repetition of actions seen. In contrast there could be marked rigidity, with resistance to any change of posture, associated with avoidance of all approaches, uncooperative behaviour or doing the opposite of what was asked.

In catatonic excitement there could be marked overactivity, talkativeness and noisiness, destructiveness and impulsive tendencies to break windows or attack others. The activity was aimless and incoherent. When marked there could be constant motor unrest and sleeplessness, a rapid failure of nutrition, epileptiform seizures and death.

The chronic catatonic condition was characterised by mannerisms. These included abnormal postures, clumsy ways of holding a spoon or fork, meaningless grimaces, odd ways of walking, such as sliding the foot back and forth two or three times before starting off, and other ceremonials for initiating movement. There was also characteristic stiffness, awkwardness, clumsiness, inaccessibility, indifference to their surroundings and general emotional dullness with outbursts for no apparent cause.

Experimental studies of motor function in schizophrenia added little to clinical studies. Shakow and Huston (Shakow & Huston 1936), for example, studied the speed of key tapping of 123 schizophrenic and 60 normal subjects in repeated sessions at 3-month intervals, and showed that the schizophrenics had a significantly slower tapping speed with more variation than the normals. This was due mainly, they felt, to their attitude and lack of co-operation. More or less every experimental study that compared the performance of schizophrenic patients and normal controls found that patients with schizophrenia perform more poorly. Lack of co-operation was the most common explanation of this.

James Chapman added a new dimension to the understanding of motor disorder in schizophrenia when he reported (Chapman 1966) on the early symptoms and the subjective experience associated with these, of a group of 40 schizophrenic patients who had been ill for between 1 and 33 months with a mean duration of illness of 11 months. They were each examined in a series of 2–12 interviews, each lasting about an hour. There was no mention of what treatment the patients had received.

Of these patients 40% showed overt and prolonged 'catatonic' behaviour. They could stay motionless for several minutes at a time in the early stages, and as the disease progressed for several hours at a time. Interestingly all these patients also reported a disturbance in visual perception, which appeared to be intricately connected with their motility:

> A 27-year-old clerk said 'Everything is all right when I stop. If I move everything I see keeps changing, everything I'm looking at gets broken up and I stop to put it together again.'

> A 24-year-old apprentice chartered accountant—'If I try to keep moving, and at the same time try to pay attention to what I see, that's when things become difficult. Normally it doesn't happen because I stop. I stop to get the depth of things, else I get the feeling I might walk into a wall. I have got to slow down to see.'

> A 20-year old apprentice turner—'When I start walking I get a fast series of pictures in front of me. Everything seems to change and revolve around me. Something goes wrong with my eyes and I've got to stop and stand still.' (Chapman 1966)

Bizarre actions or postures could be associated with visual imagery: two patients would stand still with their arms outstretched sideways, while conjuring up a memory image of Christ being crucified.

Other motor disorder was even more common—75% of the patients had experienced difficulty with movement:

> The 27-year-old clerk said—'If I do something like going for a drink of water, I've to go over each detail—find cup, walk over, turn tap, fill cup, turn tap off, drink it. I keep building up a picture. I have to change the picture each time.'

> A 19-year-old female clerk—'None of my movements come automatically to me now. I've been thinking too much about them, even walking properly, talking properly and smoking—doing anything. Before they would come automatically.'

> A 31-year-old laboratory assistant—'I don't seem to be relaxed when I'm walking. I'm thinking about it in case I might be doing it wrong and I'm trying to do it right by just trying to concentrate on every step I'm taking.'

> A 17-year-old schoolboy—'I find it very difficult to do things now, just everyday things like shaving, things that you do immediately you get up. Just things I used to do without thinking, like hanging up your coat or taking your tea. I am very easily put off now—by noises or people speaking to me. It's trying to concentrate on two things. Sometimes I have just to cut everything short and sit down. (Chapman 1966)

Observing the patients during interview, Chapman noted 'blocking phenomena' —transient periods of immobility, blank expression and fixed gaze—occurring in 95% of the 40 patients, which they could describe as 'trances', 'blank spells', 'attacks', 'stoppages of the mind' or 'dazes'.

Typically, their movements were slow, deliberate and restricted. Chapman suggested that schizophrenic patients had an impairment of the ability to carry out purposeful activities, which were previously self-regulative. They appeared to have lost access to previous learning, so that they were often unable to initiate an action simply by contemplating its goal. Instead their attention seemed to be taken up with the intermediate steps, which now required conscious co-ordination. There appeared to be a loss of the organisation normally inherent in motor activity. Given sufficient time, the schizophrenic patient might be able to carry our a single task satisfactorily. However, when required to do two or more things at the same time, for example, to move and speak or look and listen, this impairment in motor functioning became manifest.

The motor phenomena elicited by Chapman tended to be episodic and fleeting. They were seldom reported spontaneously by the patient. They were therefore easy to overlook without a special study of motor disorder.

In the last decade, Theo Manschreck and his colleagues in Boston have suggested that although motor features associated with schizophrenic disorders had often been reported, their significance had never been well understood and, since the introduction of neuroleptic medication, they had been largely neglected (Manschreck et al. 1982, Manschreck 1983). A series of studies showed that even among conservatively diagnosed schizophrenic patients, regardless of subtype, a range of abnormal motor features could be demonstrated in virtually all cases, which were not attributable to drug effects or known neurological disorder.

These disorders included spontaneous abnormalities of motor function includ-ing generalised incoordination and clumsiness; stereotypic movements—constant repetition of movements or postures, such as rubbing, nodding, grimacing; manneristic movements—odd, stylised movements or acts; motor blocking—sudden episodic reduction or cessation of movement in the middle of normal or increased activity; and abnormalities of elicited voluntary motor activity. These motor abnormalities were significantly associated with other features of their illness, such as thought disorder and affective blunting, as well as with the presence of neurological 'soft signs'. The abnormalities could be transient and missed on routine examination or casual observation if not specifically looked for.

They felt that the classic florid motor disorder of catatonia might have distracted attention from the much more common, transient and subtle features they were describing. The motor disorder was found in other psychiatric disorders but was especially prevalent in patients with schizophrenia. When it came to interpreting the significance of this motor disorder, Manschreck, while admitting that most of these disorders occurred in a variety of diseases involving basal ganglia and other sub-cortical cerebral structures, given the current lack of a neuropathology for schizophrenic disorder, fell back on a traditional psychological model based on attentional deficit. The main value of these studies was in refocussing interest on motor disorder in psychiatry, and in this they were eminently successful. Their ini-tial report in 1982 was so striking that it warranted a three-page editorial in the same issue of the journal (Marsden 1982).

FRIERN STUDY

In 1978 I studied the motor disorder of 100 patients with severe psychiatric illness (Rogers 1985). They were the 100 with the earliest dates of first admission to Friern hospital in north London who were currently patients of Richard Hunter there. By using this criterion, I hoped to select for severity of psychiatric illness, on the assumption that such patients would show the most severe motor disorder associated with psychiatric illness. Their dates of first admission to the hospital ranged from 1911 to 1955, long before Hunter joined the staff of the hospital. They all had severe persistent psychiatric disorder with an average length of current admission of over 40 years. Although the patients were not selected on the grounds of diagnosis, they had nearly all a diagnosis of schizophrenia.

These patients shed light on the historical development of the diagnosis 'schizophrenia'. The first of these patients to be admitted to Friern was in 1911, the year that Bleuler published his monograph on schizophrenia. Of the 100 patients 14, up till 1925, received the equivalent diagnosis to schizophrenia at that time in England—primary dementia. Following the English translation of Kraepelin's textbook account of dementia praecox in 1919, the diagnosis in these 14 patients became one of 'dementia praecox', for the first time in 1922. Altogether 54 of the 100 patients received a diagnosis of 'dementia praecox', for the last time in 1944. After the translation of Bleuler's textbook of schizophrenia in 1926, the diagnosis in these 54 patients became one of 'schizophrenia'. This was used for the first time in these patients in 1929. Altogether, 92 of the 100 patients subsequently received a diagnosis of 'schizophrenia'. There is hardly any other diagnosis possible for patients with prolonged, unremitting, severe psychiatric illness.

These patients were quite elderly at the time of the study. Their mean age was 72 years and the youngest was 54 years old. Their mean age on first admission to a psychiatric hospital, however, was 25 years. Their year of first admission ranged from 1907 to 1955. They were all admitted to Friern before any treatment with neuroleptic medication, which was first used in the hospital in 1954. This allowed description of motor disorder in their case notes up to 1954 to be used in the knowledge that it was definitely free of the confounding influence of such medication. Other physical treatment had been used in these patients before the introduction of neuroleptic medication but in none within 5 years of their first admission.

On current examination, the 100 patients had prominent motor disorder. This consisted of disorder of posture and tone, characteristically a tendency to flexion associated with varying degrees of rigidity and typically affecting the head and neck; disorder of motor performance, both spontaneous and elicited, character-istical difficulty with the initiation, efficient execution of, or persistence with purposive motor activity, resulting in restriction of the motor repertoire available in particular stimulus situations; disorder of motor activity, characteristically inappropriate activity, ranging from the short-lived, spontaneous and violent to the continual, stimulus-dependent and quasi-purposeful; disorder of abnormal movements, ranging from the random, simple and abrupt to the regular, complex and co-ordinated; disorder of automatic movements, such as walking and blinking; and disorder of speech production, with abnormalities reflecting those of the motor system generally.

The breakdown of motor disorder is as follows:

- *Abnormality of posture* (86%): flexion of the head when they were lying on their bed with no pillow, 72%; head flexion when upright, 63%; marked dorsal kyphosis, 37%; arm flexion, 21%; finger flexion, 21%; hyperpronation/abduction/hyperextension postures of the arms or trunk, 22%; persistence of postures, 11%.

- *Disorder of tone* (85%): increased tone in the neck, 71%; increased tone in the arms, 43%; decreased neck and arm tone, 2%; cogwheeling (regular, ratchet-like increase in tone), 45%; gegenhalten (increase in tone proportional to strength of passive movement, 8%.

- *Disorder of purposive movement* (97%): generally underactive 47%; needing help or encouragement with washing and dressing, 82%; and with eating, 26%; slowness, freezing or abruptness of movement, 21%; on request, not performing or having difficulty with pursuit eye movements, 87%; with lifting their arms, 81%, and with protruding their tongues, 66%; echopraxia, 29%.

- *Disorder of activity* (64%): general overactivity, 25%; behavioural outbursts with shouting, swearing, threatening behaviour or actual assaults, 36%; abnormal behaviours including touching or following others, touching or collecting things, self-mutilation, destroying things, stripping or excessive washing and cleaning, 20%.

- *Abnormal movements of the head, trunk or limbs* (67%): brief and random, 29%; semi-purposeful, 29%; rhythmic 26%; sustained and spasmodic, 3%; tremors, 16%; complex tics, 10%.

- *Abnormality of gait* (48%): turning their head and trunk 'in one piece', 20%; slow gait, 16%; shuffling gait, 16%; associated movements reduced, 17%; and exaggerated, 7%.

- *Abnormal spontaneous eye movements* (48%): abrupt, conjugate deviations of the eyes, 28%; roving semi-purposeful movements, 26%; staring, 3%; 'to and fro' movements, 1%.

- *Obvious abnormality of blinking* (38%): increased, 22%; decreased, rate of blinking, 14%; bursts of rapid blinking, 3%.

- *Abnormal facial movements or posture* (74%): spasmodic contractions of one or more facial muscles, 52%; fluid, random movements, mainly round the mouth, 35%; lack of facial expression, 11%; other abnormal movements of the oro-facial muscles, 9%.

- *Abnormality of speech production* (95%): practically mute, 22%; reduced speech production, 25%; outbursts of vocal activity, 53%; producing unintelligible speech, 51%; impaired volume, timbre or rate of intelligible speech, 24%; stuttering or palilalia (repetition of the last word or phrase of a sentence), 16%; echolalia, 8%.

Motor disorder in these 10 different categories had previously been noted in their case notes as part of their routine clinical assessments, as well as on current examination. Table 3.2 shows the % of patients ($n = 100$) who had some (disorder in at least one category) or a considerable amount (disorder in at least five categories) of motor disorder at different stages of their schizophrenic illnesses.

There was no striking change in the prevalence of recorded motor disorder in any of the 10 categories comparing the 34 patients whose first psychiatric admission was between 1907 and 1926, the 33 first admitted between 1927 and 1935, and the 33 first admitted between 1936 and 1955. Motor disorder was a feature of patients with severe schizophrenic illness throughout this 70-year period. This motor disorder was variable in expression: 62 of the 100 patients had had motor disorder recorded in a particular category before 1955 with no abnormality in the same category on current examination. This variability of expression of motor disorder was most marked for movement disorders and least marked for disorder of posture and purposive movement.

The patients were also assessed to discover whether a neurological diagnosis was more appropriate than a psychiatric diagnosis of schizophrenia in any of them. Eight features of possible neurological disorder were examined:

- History of possible cerebral insult before first admission.
- Abnormality on neurological examination within 5 years of first admission.
- Disorientation within 5 years of first admission.

Table 3.2 Percentage of patients with motor disorders in 10 different categories at different stages of their schizophrenic illnesses

	Disorder in at least one category (%)	Disorder in at least five categories (%)
On first admission:		
before any prolonged hospitalisation	88	10
Within 5 years of first admission:		
before any physical treatments	92	41
Prior to 1955:		
before any neuroleptic medication	98	71
On current examination	100	91

- Incontinence within 5 years of first admission.
- Fits before or after admission, excluding therapeutically induced fits.
- Abnormality of cerebro-spinal fluid, electro-encephalogram or air encephalogram on investigation.
- Diagnosis of mental subnormality.
- Diagnosis of dementia.

Altogether 86 of the 100 patients had at least one of these eight features, 25 patients had only one, 24 patients two, 22 patients three, 10 patients four, and 5 patients five of the features. These features of possible neurological disorder, therefore, were not confined to any particular subgroup among the 100 patients and, while suggestive of possible neurological disorder among a substantial proportion of the 100 patients in this study, were not sufficient to make particular neurological diagnoses in individual patients.

Thus motor disorder in these 100 contemporary patients, 92 of whom had a case note diagnosis of schizophrenia and in none of whom could an alternative neurological diagnosis be made, was very prominent and typical of that reported in patients with schizophrenia over the last 100 years. Physical treatment including neuroleptic medication was neither a necessary or sufficient cause of it.

4   Affective Disorder

CATATONIA AND AFFECTIVE DISORDER

From the outset, the catatonic motor syndrome described in the previous chapter has been associated not only with schizophrenic illnesses but with the whole spectrum of psychiatric disorders, including affective disorders. Kirby (1913) described typical catatonic symptoms in a series of patients with manic-depressive psychosis: fixed postures, hands clenched, head flexed with chin on chest, keeping the head raised from the pillow, muscular rigidity, resistance to passive movement, catalepsy, inactivity punctuated by sudden springing out of bed or impulsive striking, slowness, peculiar gait, facial abnormalities such as puckering of the lips and closure of the eyes, staring, attacks during which the eyes were rolled upwards, mutism punctuated by impulsive speech and explosive laughter.

In keeping with the psychodynamic revolution sweeping through psychiatry at the time, Kirby felt that psycho-analysis would give much valuable information regarding the nature and meaning of catatonic symptoms and suggested that stupor symbolized the death of the patient. Lange (1922) studied 700 patients with manic-depressive illness and found catatonic signs including stereotypy and catalepsy, in a quarter of them.

Stoddart was the author of a textbook of psychiatry, first published in 1908 and running to several editions (Stoddart 1926). In the section on what he still called 'melancholia' in the 1926 edition of his textbook, he described motor disturbance as the most striking and important among the physical signs in melancholia:

> The head and trunk were inclined forwards as in paralysis agitans and there was slight flexion of the hips and knees. There was also slight flexion of the shoulders and the elbows, held rigidly to the side, flexed to a right angle. The corners of the mouth were turned down and the forehead wrinkled from contraction of the frontalis or corrugator muscles or both. There was rigidity affecting the large proximal joints most, and with the rigidity slight weakness of the affected muscles. All movements were slow. In stupor there was no movement. Superficial reflexes were reduced. There could be nystagmoid jerking on extreme lateral deviation of the eyes and weakness of accommodation. Phonation was weak, lower pitched than in health and monotonous with poor articulation. Speech was reduced and in stupor absent. There was slowness in reacting to questions and answering them. In stupor, the extremities could be blue, swollen and oedematous. In agitated melancholia, there was constant movement, pacing about, walking, not from the hips, but from the ankles and knees, wringing the hands, picking pieces of skin from the fingers or face, or fumbling with buttons. In mania, the state of motor excitement affected mainly the

large proximal joints, the trunk swaying freely on walking with exaggerated movements at the hips on running. Elbows were typically abducted from the side. Superficial reflexes were exaggerated (Stoddart 1926).

In the preface to this 1926 fifth edition, however, he gives an insight into the conceptual changes that had overtaken psychiatry since the first edition in 1908:

> When the manual was first published, my endeavour was to induce the reader to think neurologically of mental processes, normal and morbid, and to study them from a neurological point of view. Since that time, however, owing to the psychological researches of Freud, and previously Janet and others, it has been found that we gain a clearer insight into mental processes when we approach them from a purely psychological standpoint (Stoddart 1926).

In the United States, where the swing to psychodynamic psychiatry was more complete than in most other countries, catatonia was not considered part of affective disorder and only included as a subtype of schizophrenia in DSM-I, DSM-II, and DSM-III. Until a few years ago, it was still indexed as such in virtually all US psychiatric textbooks (Ries 1985).

More recently, this position has changed with a series of papers re-affirming the non-specific nature of the catatonic syndrome and suggesting that affective disorder represents by far and away the largest non-schizophrenic psychiatric catatonic group, and there have even been suggestions that catatonic signs are seen most frequently in patients with diagnosable affective disorders, especially mania. Studying the phenomenology of 52 patients who satisfied research criteria for mania, but who had been given other diagnoses, mainly schizophrenia, Taylor and Abrams (Taylor & Abrams 1973) found catatonic symptoms in 13.5%. The same authors (Taylor & Abrams 1977) later considered 123 patients who had been admitted over a 14-month period to two acute-treatment in-patient psychiatric units with bipolar affective disorder. They found that 28% had had two or more of the following catatonic signs: stereotypy, posturing, catalepsy, automatic obedience, negativism, echolalia/echopraxia or stupor; which were pronounced and persisted for at least a period of hours. These 28% did not differ from the rest of the affective patients in demographic characteristics, psychopathology, family history or treatment response. When they examined (Abrams & Taylor 1976) 55 patients, admitted over the same period, who showed one or more of the following catatonic signs: mutism, stereotypy, posturing, catalepsy, automatic obedience, negativism, echolalia/echopraxia, or stupor; 62% satisfied criteria for mania, 9% for depression, 7% for schizophrenia and 5% for reactive psychosis, while 16% were diagnosed as having cerebral disorder.

In 1986, Barnes and colleagues (Barnes et al. 1986) presented their accumulated experience of 25 cases of the catatonic syndrome seen in one neurological unit between 1972 and 1984. They defined catatonia as at least catalepsy, posturing or waxy flexibility in combination with one of the following: mutism, negativism, impulsiveness, grimacing, stereotypies, mannerisms, command automatism, echopraxia/echolalia or verbigeration. They found that nine patients (36%) had an affective illness, five patients had an organic cause and one patient had schizophrenia. In 10 patients (40%) no psychiatric or organic cause could be determined despite intensive investigation.

In a series of studies, Guenther and colleagues (Guenther et al. 1988), quoting in their introduction the work of Wernicke and Kleist, have shown what they call a 'psychotic motor syndrome' both in schizophrenic and depressed patients, consisting of disturbance of oro-facial movement, fine and gross movements of the dominant hand and complex motor co-ordination of the extremities. This syndrome was found in 'endogenous' depressed patients, both unipolar and bipolar, but not in healthy controls or non-endogenous depressed patients. It was present in both medicated and unmedicated patients and there was no evidence that the motor syndrome was secondary to anti-psychotic medication. The authors could not demonstrate any difference between the syndrome in schizophrenic and depressed patients, suggesting that it might represent the same alteration of cerebral function in both groups. In contrast to schizophrenic patients, who showed the motor syndrome both on presentation and in clinical remission, however, the depressed patients showed complete disappearance of the motor syndrome on clinical recovery.

PSYCHOMOTOR RETARDATION IN DEPRESSION

Although any catatonic motor disorder can be associated with affective illness, the component that is especially associated with depressive disorder, is psychomotor retardation or slowing of cognitive and motor function. Psychomotor retardation is the most consistent feature characterising major depression or melancholia (Nelson & Charney 1981). Clinical descriptions of it have been consistent over the last 60 years. Compare the accounts of Bleuler (Bleuler 1923) and Widlocher (Widlocher 1983):

> All psychical activity is slowed. The association of ideas is retarded. Thinking becomes slow and laborious, revolving monotonously about the patient's misfortune. Movements require just as much exertion as thinking. The limbs are as heavy as lead. Movements become effortful, slow and weak. A patient might want to change her place at table, lift up the chair, and then require half an hour to decide whether and where she should place it. In more severe cases even retardation of sensory perception can be demonstrated (Bleuler 1923).

> There is a general slowing down of motor activity in limbs and trunk. The patient rarely moves his trunk or limbs, especially proximally. The amplitude of movements is reduced. In stupor, there is almost no movement. The shoulders droop and the patient stares towards the floor. The gait is impaired, with smaller, shuffling steps and loss of associated movements. The face is immobile and blank. Speech is slowed with a weak, monotonous voice. Psychic activity is slowed. Responses are slow and brief. There is impoverishment of ideas, with ruminative thinking, and difficulty

moving to a new idea. There is difficulty with concentration and memory, due to impaired recall. Motor and mental slowing are generally felt as fatigue, distressing in everyday life and not improved and even worsened by rest. Not all activity is affected equally. It can vary through the day, typically worse early in the morning. It is environmentally sensitive (Widlocher 1983).

Interpretations of the cause of this slowing, however, have varied substantially. In 1934, Aubrey Lewis published a historical review of melancholia (Lewis 1934a) and a clinical survey of depressive states based on a detailed study of cases he had examined at the Maudsley hospital (Lewis 1934b). These two papers set the seal on our modern concept of depression. Melancholia had been a category of mental disorder since the Greeks, with various connotations. By the end of the nineteenth century, the term meant a psychosis whose chief symptoms were a primary sad change of mood and a primary slowing of ideation or inhibition of thought. Some, such as Wernicke, attributed a predominant significance to the retardation of thought, but gradually affective change came to be regarded as its central feature. In 1904, Adolph Meyer suggested applying the term depression to the whole class of melancholia, and this became generally accepted. Lewis felt that this development was fully justified.

With respect to psychomotor slowing, Lewis noted that although all writers agreed as to its importance in depression, few defined it or its manifestations, leaving the name to speak for itself. He considered retardation in the 61 patients with depressive states he examined, under the headings of thinking and action. As regards subjective change in thinking, many complained of a constant surge of thoughts, but none that their thoughts seemed slower or fewer. On examination, he felt that inattention and preoccupation seemed responsible for most of their deficiencies, for example, with tests of memory, grasp and calculation. As regards action, fatigue or inertia was reported by the patients or their relatives in all but two of the cases. On examination, however, the incapacity for action was greater in the patients' reports than it appeared in their behaviour. What the patient appreciated as difficulty in thinking could strike the observer as slowness in performing an operation, though actual slowing of movement was less characteristic than incapacity to complete a task. Retardation, or definite slowing of movement and occasionally of talk, or evidence of inhibition, as recognised in speech broken off before completion, was present in 19 of the 61 cases. Stupor, the extreme form of retardation, with complete or almost complete failure to react to external stimuli and immobility, was found at some stage in five of the patients, and a less definite form or semi-stupor in a further six patients.

At this time, psychological explanations of this slowing were common. Views such as McCurdy's (McCurdy 1925) were typical. Painful thoughts are slow and retardation was an expression of mental pain. Some authors continued, like Wernicke in the previous century, to suggest a primary role for slowing. Harriet Babcock the psychologist (Babcock 1933), hypothesised that abnormal slowness among psychotic patients could account almost entirely for their general cognitive impairment. Indeed, she believed that much of their general behaviour, such as unsociability, could be explained in terms of this relatively specific defect. She showed that a large number of very simple motor and mental speed tests differentiated well between normal and psychotic subjects.

Shapiro and Nelson (Shapiro & Nelson 1955) set out to test Babcock's theory in different psychiatric disorders, including depression. They compared 20 normal subjects, 20 neurotics, 20 manic–depressives, 20 schizophrenics and 20 organics on a variety of neuropsychological tests, including the Nufferno speed tests, which measured cognitive speed by measuring the time taken to correctly solve problems that could be solved by 80% of the population. They concluded that psychiatric illness was associated with apparent impairment of all the cognitive functions they examined. All types of cognitive measures differentiated between normal, neurotic and psychotic patients whose illnesses were of long duration, but they were unable to differentiate between brain-damaged and chronic schizophrenic patients. Slowness was the most important of all the variables they examined because it differentiated most powerfully between normal and abnormal groups. When subjects were matched for their scores on tests of vocabulary, problem solving and memory for new word definitions, psychomotor slowness still differentiated between normal and abnormal groups. When, however, the opposite was done and relatively normal and abnormal groups were matched for scores on the psychomotor speed test, then tests of vocabulary, problem solving and memory for the definition of new words did not differentiate significantly between the groups. Slowness on psychomotor speed tests correlated more highly and more consistently with independent subjective estimates of severity of illness than any of the other tests. The slowness could not be accounted for by sedation since the most heavily sedated patients were not necessarily the slowest, and non-sedated patients were still significantly slower than normal subjects. Like Babcock, Shapiro and Nelson suggested that this slowness of function might be a primary component of psychiatric disorder.

These results were confirmed by others but with a different interpretation. Payne and Hewlett (Payne & Hewlett 1960), for example, found that motor, mental and perceptual speed tests differentiated depressive and normal subjects but this was because patients with profound depression could not free their minds from feelings of guilt and unworthiness and so were unable to attend and concentrate. Distraction was the main cause of their abnormal cognitive slowness.

Shapiro and Nelson (Shapiro & Nelson 1955), reviewed 11 studies of reaction time in psychiatric patients before 1955, varying from simple visuo-motor to multiple choice reaction time. The studies varied considerably in experimental and statistical sophistication, but their outcome was sufficiently unanimous to warrant Bevan–Lewis' original finding in 1890 that all types of fully co-operative psychiatric patients showed a decided prolongation of reaction times compared to normals. Hall and Stride (Hall & Stride 1952) studied reaction time latency to an auditory stimulus in 20 normal subjects, 40 'neurotic' patients, 40 depressives and 25 schizophrenics. The neurotics and depressives were subdivided into two matched-age groups of under and over 40 years of age. In the under 40s, normal subjects were more consistent and quicker in response than the neurotic group, and these quicker than the depressives. The difference between neurotics and depressives was accentuated in the over 40s. The schizophrenics had the longest reaction times. A number of patients were re-tested at various stages in the course of their illness. In general, patients with prolonged reaction times who improved clinically showed a significant quickening of reaction time, whereas patients who did not improve clinically continued to have similar or even longer reaction times. Martin and Rees (Martin & Rees 1966) again found that depressives had a slower mean reaction time than the control group, and that this objective measure of slowness was closely related to clinically observed retardation. Many were slow to grasp instructions and said they had difficulty in summoning the required effort. They showed that when the patients were told that their responses were slow and urged to try again, they could improve considerably.

Friedman (Friedman 1964), in a study comparing a sample of 55 depressives and 65 normal subjects, matched for sex, age, education and brief estimate of intellectual level, seemed to show that depression was not associated with any significant cognitive disorder. On 82 test scores of 33 cognitive, perceptual and psychomotor tests, the depressives were impaired on only three at the $p = 0.01$ level of significance and six at the $p = 0.05$ level. Weckowicz et al. (1972), however, criticised Friedman for not separating 'speed' tests from 'power' tests. Most of the tests on which Friedman's depressive patients performed worse than controls were in fact those related to speed of performance. Weckowicz investigated the relation of speed of performance on motor, perceptual and cognitive tasks, to depressive illness and age. He compared 30 newly admitted female depressed patients scoring more than 20 on Beck's depression inventory and 30 female volunteers, matched for social and educational background, none of whom had a depression inventory score greater than 12. Both groups were divided into three age groups (15–29, 30–44 and 45–59 years) and matched for age. Altogether 24 tests were used: six to measure level of cognitive functioning and 18 to measure speed of performance on a variety of tasks. Age affected the speed of cognitive and motor functioning to a greater extent than scores of 'power' tests. The depressed patients tended to show a lower performance speed than normal subjects of comparable age. The combined effects of age and depression on speed of performance tended to be additive. Only one test consistently differentiated the effect of depression from that of age, the simple reaction time, which was significantly longer in depressive patients, irrespective of age. When he came to interpret the results of this elegant study, however, Weckowicz could only suggest that the poor performance on speed tests of depressed and older subjects was due to 'complex motivational factors'.

Cornell et al. (1984) attempted to assess the relative contribution of cognitive and motor factors in psychomotor response times with a series of tests where the cognitive demand varied but the motor demand remained the same. They compared 14 'melancholic', 14 'non-melancholic' depressed patients and 14 normal controls. The patients were drug-free for at least 7 days. Stimuli were presented on a video screen and the response was the pressing of one of two standard push-buttons with the preferred hand. Response times for all four tests were longer in both patient groups compared to the controls, and longer in the melancholic compared to the non-melancholic patients. The results suggested a motor component of the psychomotor retardation in both melancholic and non-melancholic depressive patients, with a cognitive component in the melancholic group.

Gietke et al. (1981) compared the 'cognitive' auditory evoked potential (P3) latency and reaction times to infrequent clicks in 13 patients with primary depressive illness compared to 13 healthy aged-matched controls. Reaction times were significantly longer in the depressed patients, but neither P3 latency nor P3 amplitude differed between the groups. They concluded that the delayed reaction times in the depressed patients must be due to impaired selection activation or execution of the motor response rather than stimulus evaluation. Brand and Jolles (1987), using four versions of Sternberg's memory comparison tasks, found that depressive patients showed slower scanning than controls and other patient groups as well as slowing on the non-scanning stages of information processing. Knott and Lapierre (1987) examined cortical evoked potentials and the integrated electromyogram from the dominant forearm extensor muscles during psychomotor task performance in 21 women with significant depressive illness and 21 controls. The depressed patients showed an overall slower reaction time than the controls and analysis of this showed that both central processing time and motor response time contributed to this slowing. No correlation between these measures and depression severity, as assessed by Hamilton rating, was found. No clinical assessment of retardation was carried out.

With colleagues at the National Hospital, Queen Square (Rogers et al. 1987), I found both cognitive and motor slowing in the performance of a computerised digit symbol substitution test in 30 patients with primary depressive illness, compared to age- and education-matched normal control subjects. Use of a simpler cognitive task, a matched-choice reaction time test involving the same motor responses, allowed estimation of the relative contributions of motor and cognitive elements in the digit symbol test. On re-testing 12 patients and 12 of the normal controls after an average of 6 months, the patients, who were on anti-depressant medication throughout, showed significant improvement in both their depression and response time for the digit symbol test, due mainly to improvement in cognitive slowing.

The depressed patients also showed a significant clinical motor impairment compared to the normal controls at the start of the study with a significant improvement on re-testing. The motor impairment was measured with the Webster rating scale, normally used to assess the severity of parkinsonism. It consists of 10 items—bradykinesia of hands, rigidity, posture, upper extremity swing, gait, tremor, facies, seborrhoea, speech and self-care—with a score of 0–3 for each item, giving a total motor impairment score for the 10 items out of 30. The mean score of the normal controls was 0 with a range of 0–2. The mean score of 30 untreated patients with Parkinson's disease, tested in the same study, was 12 with a range of 3–21. The mean score of the patients with primary depression was 5 with a range of 0–13. The highest rating of 13 was in a patient emerging from stupor. The difference between parkinsonian and depressed patients and between depressed patients and normal controls were both significant at the $p < 0.001$ level. Each of the 10 individual items contributed to the rating in the depressed patients, with the highest ratings for arm swing, facial expression and speech impairment. The only items with a mean rating per patient in the parkinsonian group of over twice that in the depressed group were tremor, rigidity, self-care and bradykinesia.

Two of the 30 consecutively referred depressed patients were taking neuroleptic medication at the time of testing. This might, conventionally, have been thought to contribute significantly to their Webster rating and thus to vitiate the use of this rating in their cases. Further analysis, however, shows that the contribution of neuroleptic medication to their motor disorder was not straightforward. One was the patient in stupor. When she was re-tested out of stupor on the same dose of neuroleptic her Webster score had markedly improved. The second patient was initially admitted to a neurological ward at the National Hospital for investigation and, before the diagnosis became clear, was noted by the admitting doctor to have a resting tremor, increased tone and difficulty initiating movements. At this time, his only medication was a benzodiazepine. By the time he was tested, treatment for his depressive psychosis with an anti-depressant and neuroleptic had been started, with improvement in both his depressive symptoms and motor signs.

Schlegel et al. (1988) correlated ratings for depression on a variety of different scales and measurements on computed tomography (CT) brain scan in 44 patients with a major depressive episode, controlling for age-related CT changes. The common psychopathological features of the scales, which correlated with measures of mild brain atrophy, were psychomotor retardation and emotional blunting. The highest correlations of all were between different atrophy measures and the retardation items on one of the scales, the Bech–Rafaelson Melancholia Scale. Recent investigations of affective disorders (Kupfer et al. 1974) have suggested that changes in psychomotor activity occur very early in the course of these disorders, before psychological symptoms are prominent, and tend to persist after obvious mood changes recede, thus being more useful than the mood changes in following the clinical course of the illnesses.

Although mood disturbance has been regarded as the primary psychopathological expression of affective disorder since the change in prevailing paradigm in psychiatry at the turn of the century, there is in fact no evidence that psychomotor and cognitive disturbances in these disorders are secondary to feelings of sadness or elation. Widlocher (1983) points the way forward when he suggests re-establishing psychomotor retardation as a primary disturbance and the central feature of affective disorder as opposed to mood disturbance, as was already suggested last century.

BRADYPHRENIA IN PARKINSON'S DISEASE

Both catatonic motor disorder and psychomotor retardation are not specific for any particular psychiatric disorder, and form part of accepted neurological disorders. Although this is accepted in principal, the full extent of the overlap between the same motor disorders present in psychiatric and neurological disorders has been clouded by the historical division of neurology and psychiatry resulting in the separate vocabularies for neurological and psychiatric motor disorders, described in the first two chapters. This is well illustrated by the separate development of the concepts of psychomotor retardation in depression and bradyphrenia in parkinsonism.

The term 'bradyphrenia' was coined by the French neurologist, Naville in 1922 (Naville 1922) to describe what he felt was a new psychiatric syndrome produced by the epidemic of encephalitis lethargica, which had swept across Europe (Rogers 1986). Bradyphrenia meant slowing of mental function but the syndrome was much wider than this, including impairment of attention, interest, initiative and the capacity for sustained effort and work. There was lethargy of thought, movement and affect. Cognitive functioning was slowed but intelligence was spared except for a slight impairment of memory. An expressionless face was typical. Naville described bradyphrenia as a loss of psychic tone. Those severely affected became uncommunicative and did nothing without constant prompting. In its extreme form, there could be complete loss of psychomotor activity. Naville speculated about a special psychomotor system whose physiology awaited elucidation.

A similar syndrome had been previously described in idiopathic Parkinson's disease and the similarity to psychomotor retardation in depressive illness noted:

> An invisible weight seems to crush the intellect and slow down perception, movement and ideas . . . The present case is obviously one of paralysis agitans with dementia, but one cannot help, on observing these symptoms, but think of certain cases of melancholic stupor, such as one sees in our mental asylums (Ball 1882).

Benjamin Ball was France's first professor of psychiatry but because of the splitting of the ways between neurology and psychiatry shortly after Ball was writing, the overlap between Parkinson's disease and depressive illness, which struck him, has only recently been taken up again as a focus of interest. Of interest too is Ball's use of the term 'dementia' to describe slowing of cognitive functioning as part of the parkinsonian syndrome. We now use the term 'sub-cortical dementia' to describe this, after its introduction by Albert in the 1970s (Albert et al. 1974).

Naville did not clearly distinguish bradyphrenia from the still evolving concept of akinesia. In the patients with bradyphrenia he described, peripheral execution of movement could be slow and there could be a delay between the impulse for movement and the start of its execution, but what was especially slow was the impulse for movement. At times, movements could be performed correctly, which at other times were completely impossible—what came to be known as kinesia paradoxica. Akinesia only slowly became accepted as a major motor component of the parkinsonian syndrome after the epidemic encephalitis. Up till then, akinesia, like bradyphrenia, was considered as a psychiatric syndrome (Ajuriaguerra 1975). When akinesia became fully established in the 1960s, bradyphrenia became regarded as its mental corollary and renamed 'psychic akinesia'.

Naville felt that the syndrome of bradyphrenia he was describing had implications for the relationship of motor and mental phenomena in a wide range of disorders including depressive illness. Economo (1931) described similarities between bradyphrenia and depression following epidemic encephalitis. Both could show diurnal variation, being better in the evening. When bradyphrenia was severe it could produce a degree of psychomotor retardation commonly associated with the cataleptic states of psychoses, such as depressive stupor. Hans Steck, in his study of the mental sequelae of the encephalitis (Steck 1931), distinguished different post-encephalitic depressive syndromes, contrasting neurasthenia-like states that could lead onto bradyphrenia, and melancholic states with tearfulness, ideas of guilt and suicide, and hypochondriasis.

After the introduction of levodopa for the treatment of Parkinson's disease in the 1960s, there was renewed interest in the relationship of parkinsonism and depression. A series of studies found a prevalence of depression higher in parkinsonian patients than in matched control groups, independent of degree of disability, the duration of the illness and medication. The idea began to gain ground of an overlap between the physiological mechanisms underlying both Parkinson's disease and depression. Ajuriaguerra (1971) studied 204 patients with parkinsonism and found depressive states in 70%. Like Steck, he divided these depressive states into two types: 60% of his cases had 'simple' depressive states, characterised by some sadness but mainly by lack of drive and fatiguability; a further 10% had more severe depressive symptoms or 'melancholia', with ideas of guilt, suicide and hypochondriasis. All the patients with simple depression had significant akinesia and levodopa could produce a parallel improvement in motor and affective disorder. In the group with melancholia, levodopa produced a significant improvement in motor disorder with less effect on the depressive symptoms, requiring the addition of a tricyclic anti-depressant.

An overlap of motor features of affective disorder and parkinsonism, such as size of handwriting, was also noted. Court (1964) administered a battery of tests, including four writing tasks, to 44 consecutively admitted acute psychiatric patients and at intervals during their stay, and to 34 normal controls. Quite considerable changes in the size of handwriting were associated with changes in mood, decrease in size being related to depressive states and increase related to states of excitement. The size of writing increased as patients who had been depressed improved in mood; conversely patients who were in states of excitement on admission produced smaller writing as they improved clinically.

Several authors tried the effect of levodopa on depressive illness, and found that it had a therapeutic effect of depression with motor retardation, without otherwise being an effective anti-depressant (Goodwin et al. 1970, Matussek et al. 1970, Kanzler & Malitz 1972). Van Praag et al. (1975) studied central dopamine metabolism in various disorders, including depression and parkinsonism, by means of the probenicid technique to measure dopamine metabolites in cerebro-spinal fluid. They concluded that decreased dopamine metabolism was associated with hypomotility rather than being specific for any particular disease or syndrome, and that this decreased dopamine turnover was related to the cause of the hypomotility rather than simply being its consequence. Banki (1977), in another cerebro-spinal fluid study of depressive illness, showed that dopamine turnover, as measured by homovallinic acid concentration, was reduced in depressed patients with retardation but not in those without. The implication of all these studies was that there was a close relationship between akinesia, bradyphrenia and the psychomotor retardation of depressive illness, with impairment of dopamine function as a common pathological factor.

Price et al. (1978) found a marked decrease in dopamine levels in certain parts of the limbic forebrain in parkinsonian patients' brains at post-mortem, and suggested that this might be an important factor in the aetiology of affective disorder in Parkinson's disease. Javoy-Agid & Agid (1980) demonstrated lesions of the meso-cortico-limbic dopaminergic projection system in the brains of patients who had suffered from Parkinson's disease, and suggested that these might play a role both in the motor akinesia and cognitive disorder of this disease. Agid et al. (1984) suggested that involvement of the meso-cortico-limbic dopaminergic system in parkinsonism was the basis of bradyphrenia and depression in this condition, which were often closely associated. Lesions of a single projection system innervating several areas with different functions would explain this association. Loss of dopaminergic innervation to the pre-frontal cortex could be responsible for bradyphrenia and explain its similarity to frontal lobe syndromes, and loss of innervation to limbic cortex the basis for affective disorder.

In our study of psychomotor retardation in depression and bradyphrenia in Parkinson's disease (Rogers et al. 1987) we used, as Naville had originally done, tests of differing cognitive difficulty requiring the same motor response, but now with computerised testing. We tested the performance of 30 patients with Parkinson's disease, matched for age and education with the 30 patients with depressive illness and the 30 normal controls, before starting any dopaminergic treatment. Cognitive processing time was significantly increased in the parkinsonian patients, but only in those with significant depressive symptoms. On re-testing 12 of the parkinsonian patients after starting dopaminergic treatment, the most significant association with improvement in response time for the cognitive test used was improvement in their depression rating, suggesting an association between cognitive slowing and depression in parkinsonian patients.

This study, like the others reviewed, suggest that bradyphrenia in parkinsonism and psychomotor retardation in depressive illness might be similar or identical clinical phenomena viewed from two different perspectives. Until fairly recently, authors were keen to distance themselves from a neurological interpretation of psychomotor retardation. Kiloh (1961), for example, writing in 1961 on 'pseudo-dementia' in psychiatric illness, and notably depression, warned against clinical features of retardation such as a slow shuffling gait, which could create the illusion of involvement of the central nervous system. This should now be a thing of the past. The overlap of psychomotor retardation, which has good claim to be the central clinical feature of depressive illness, with features of known neurological disease, such as bradyphrenia in parkinsonism, should be the focus of intensive study.

5 Obsessive-Compulsive Disorder, Hysteria and Mental Handicap

OBSESSIVE-COMPULSIVE DISORDER

Obsessions are defined as recurrent, persistent ideas, thoughts, images, or impulses that are experienced as involuntary, senseless or repugnant. Attempts are made to ignore or suppress them. Compulsions are repetitive and seemingly purposeful behaviours that are performed according to certain rules or in a stereotyped fashion. The act is performed with a sense of subjective compulsion often coupled with a desire to resist the compulsion, which is usually recognised as senseless behaviour.

The history of neurological views of obsessive-compulsive disorder (OCD) has been well reviewed by Nigel Hymas (Hymas & Prasad 1989), and this section draws heavily from this account. As with the psychiatric conditions already dealt with, obsessive-compulsive disorders underwent a swing in prevalent explanatory paradigm, from neurological to psychological, over the last decade of the nineteenth century and has undergone a swing back again starting in the 1960s. Again there was a transient revival of neurological interest in obsessive-compulsive disorder in the wake of the epidemic encephalitis in the 1920s and 30s, with most of this work 'forgotten' in the recent re-awakening of interest in neurological features of obsessive-compulsive disorder.

Janet, whose clinical descriptions of the disorder at the turn of the century (Janet 1903) remain unsurpassed, played a large part in establishing the predominance of the new psychological paradigm but he, like Freud, believed that psychological formulations were merely the best that could be done with the currently available knowledge, and would eventually give way to neurological formulations. Subsequent generations, however, forgot this aspiration, lost interest in neurology and became solely interested in psychological function divorced from cerebral function. Until recently, absence of demonstrable brain disease formed part of the definition of obsessive-compulsive disorder.

Obsessive-compulsive disorder was a well-known accompaniment to post-encephalitic parkinsonism (Economo 1931). Claude and his colleagues, reporting three cases of post-encephalitic obsessional behaviour (Claude et al. 1927a), discussed its neurological implications in terms forward-looking even for today:

> ...we see in our patients a classical picture of obsessional illness. Thus, as well as the anatomic-clinical syndromes of a focal nature such as are seen in neurology, and

for which one reserves the term organic, one must allow the presence of diffuse, fluctuating and widespread processes affecting diverse areas of the brain, giving rise to functional disorder which, if it persists, can lead to lasting anatomical changes (Claude et al. 1927).

This line of thinking, however, was only taken up by a few such as Brickner et al. (1940), who suggested that obsessive-compulsive states should be considered as part of a continuum of different disorders, the common feature of which was 'repetitiveness or fixedness of action dominating the intellectual or muscular picture'.

Such repetitive or fixed behaviour, when clinically observed in the strictly psychological (neuro-intellectual) domain is ordinarily thought of as obsessive. In the psychomotor field it is called compulsive, and in the strictly motor sphere it has a variety of names, depending largely on the syndrome in which it appears— perseveration, catatonia, propulsion, iteration, echolalia, palilalia, stereotypy of movement or thoughts and others. Indeed, if examples leading from perseveration to obsessive thinking are presented in sequence, it is difficult to make a fundamental distinction between any two of them. The uniform thread of repetitiveness or fixedness which runs through all of these suggests that a common physiological mechanism may underlie them all, regardless of the behaviour field in which they are clinically manifest (Brickner et al. 1940).

Schilder (1938), because of his experiences with post-encephalitic obsessional disorder put forward a neurological explanation of idiopathic obsessive-compulsive disorder. He felt that motor disorder in cases of obsessional disorder with no history of encephalitis was common, and that about one-third of these showed such features, including rigidity of the face, mask-like facies, flexor rigidity of the arms, tremor, impaired eye convergence, great urge to talk and propulsive features in speech, hyperactivity and 'motor urges of a higher degree'. Vujic (1952) agreed with Schilder. He described a number of abnormal motor signs in a wide variety of neurotic conditions, particularly obsessional illness where he felt signs of abnormal posture of the arms and hands, at rest and when outstretched, narrowing of the palpebral fissure, tonic contraction of the frontalis muscle and loss of arm swing walking, complemented those of Schilder.

The 1980s saw an increasing interest in neurological features of obsessive-compulsive disorder (OCD). Denckla (1989), for example, reported neurological abnormality in 81% of 54 children and adolescents with OCD, including choreiform movements in 24%. Hollander et al. (1990) reported the first comprehensive, controlled study of neurological soft signs in adult patients with OCD. They found significant abnormalities in total number of soft signs, fine motor co-ordination and involuntary movements in 41 patients aged 18–53 years meeting DSM-III criteria for OCD compared to 20 matched normal controls aged 21–60 years old. The patients had no focal neurological disorder or major medical illness and all had been medication-free for at least two weeks. It was found that 95% of the 41 patients had at least one abnormal soft sign and abnormalities in fine motor co-ordination occurred in 83%, with involuntary movements in 32%.

Rachman (1974) described 10 patients with severe slowness in the execution of simple tasks of daily living, such as dressing, bathing or eating. He described the patients as resembling a 'slow motion movie' and called the syndrome primary obsessional slowness. His explanation of the syndrome was still in psychological terms of 'meticulousness'. Hymas et al. (1991) examined 17 of 59 consecutive referrals to the Behaviour Therapy Unit of the Maudsley Hospital who had 'slowing' as a significant feature of their symptomatology. Typical symptoms were having to take several hours over everyday activities such as eating, dressing, washing or bathing. These 17 had higher obsessionality ratings than the rest of the group: two had associated psychiatric disorder (Asberger's syndrome and depression) and four had associated neurological disorder (Parkinson's disease in two and Tourette syndrome in two). All had a normal CT brain scan. None suffered from major depression.

The following features were assessed—speech, posture, elicited movements of head, neck and face, alternating, sequential and skilled upper limb movements, writing, repetitive lower limb movements, whole body movements and gait—as well as a standard neurological examination. A matched normal control group was also assessed. The patients showed subtle neurological abnormalities compared to the healthy controls, including loss of motor fluency, hesitancy of initiation of limb movements, speech and gait abnormalities, cogwheel rigidity, complex repetitive movements and tics. They showed significant impairment on almost all aspects of motor function examined. Their slowness was mainly due to difficulty initiating goal-directed action and suppressing intrusive and perseverative behaviour. They resembled the cases described by Rachman with a meticulous concern to do things properly, periods of motionlessness and slow motion of the limbs, and the breakdown of ordinary behaviour into its component movements with prolongation of each component.

The authors suggested that obsessional slowness might represent dysfunction of the frontal–basal–ganglia loop system (Alexander 1986). This was supported by a study of positron emission tomography in some of those patients demonstrating bilaterally increased oxygen metabolism at rest in orbital frontal, pre-motor and mid-frontal cortex (Sawle et al. 1991). This, it was suggested, was related to the patients' difficulty with internal preparation for movement, which was comparable to the difficulties shown in response preparation and response inhibition by patients with chronic medial frontal lobe lesions (Verfaellie & Heilman 1987).

Obsessive-compulsive disorder has significant associations with other motor disorder and notably tics. Tics are recurrent, involuntary, repetitive, rapid, purposeless movements. In his classic monograph on tics, Meige (1905) described them as a psychomotor disturbance. He noted the frequent association of tics with obsessional states, and considered that lack of cortical control was important in the development of both phenomena. The appearance of both tics and obsessive-compulsive phenomena as post-encephalitic phenomena following encephalitis a prompted renewed speculation about the relationship between them. o (1931) saw the neurological implications of this association:

> . . . compulsive movements may also contain psychological elements which associate themselves with the originally organic motor disturbances and increase them to compulsive actions . . . in these chronic disturbances of motility we find the patient saying, not, as we have seen in certain acute disturbances of motility, 'I have a twitch in my hand', but rather as a rule, 'I have got to move my hand that way'. The frequent subjectivisation of these processes, experienced as compulsory by the patient . . . is, I believe, one of their characteristic attributes (Economo 1931).

The Tourette syndrome, first described by Gilles de la Tourette (1885), is defined by the criteria of age of onset between 2 and 15 years, tics affecting multiple muscle groups, vocal tics, ability to suppress the movements voluntarily for minutes to hours, variation in the intensity of the symptoms over weeks to months and duration of more than one year. Coprolalia (compulsive swearing) and echo phenomena (compulsive imitation) can be associated features. Many authors have reported a significant association with obsessional disorder. Obsessional symptoms, traits or illness have been reported with a prevalence of between 11 and 80% of patients with Tourette syndrome in different studies, and are correlated with coprolalia and echo phenomena in these patients (Rogers 1989; Trimble 1989).

Some authors (Yaryura-Tobias 1983) have suggested regarding Tourette syndrome as an obsessive-compulsive disorder. Cummings & Frankel (1985) examined the similarities between these two disorders, including age of onset, life-long course, waxing and waning of symptoms, involuntary and intrusive 'ego-alien' behaviour and experience, occurrence in the same families, and worsening with depression and anxiety. Pitman et al. (1987) compared 16 patients with Tourette syndrome, 16 with obsessive-compulsive disorder and 16 normal controls: they found that six of the patients with OCD and one of the normal controls had tics, and that the tics in the OCD group were similar to those seen in the Tourette group. Pauls et al. (1986) have shown a genetic relationship between Tourette syndrome and obsessive-compulsive disorder.

Obsessive-compulsive disorder is a disorder of behaviour. In cerebral terms, there is no sharp distinction between behaviour and motor disorder, and obsessive-compulsive disorder could be regarded neurologically as a motor disorder.

HYSTERIA

The diagnosis of hysteria includes several distinct concepts. It can refer to a personality type, a polysymptomatic disorder and so-called conversion symptoms or 'neurological hysteria'. All three can be present by themselves or in any combination in the same patient.

Conversion symptoms are unexplained symptoms suggesting neurological disease. They can affect either sex and patients of any age, and they are often associated with other physical or psychiatric disorders. They can be precipitated by stress, typically in war time, and symptoms often include motor disorder. Analysing 381 cases, Ljungeberg (1957) found that the commonest presentations were with gait disturbance (47%), fits (20%), tremor (10%) and paralysis (10%). Catatonic signs have also been reported in conversion hysteria (Gelenberg 1976). Features distinguishing hysterical from 'genuine' neurological disorder are abrupt onset, static course, spontaneous remissions, remissions with psychotherapy, complexity making them unclassifiable, absence of other neurological signs, inconsistency, with ability to perform some functions despite severe symptoms, changing characteristics, increase with attention, lessening with distractibility, unresponsiveness to neurological medication and responsiveness to placebo (Koller et al. 1989). Another feature of hysterical disorder is its failure to comply with orthodox neurological dysfunction, as in 'wrong-way' deviation of the tongue towards the normal side in hysterical hemiparesis and deviation of the eyes away from the examiner in pseudoseizures (Keane 1986, Armon 1991).

Analysis of these disorders has not advanced beyond simple description. In a study of 60 cases of hysterical gait disorder, Keane (1989) described hemiparetic, paraparetic, ataxic, trembling, dystonic, truncal myoclonus, stiff-legged (robot), slapping (tabetic) and camptocormia (bent back) varieties. In 1918, Roussy and Lhermitte had described astasia–abasia, pseudotabetic, pseudopolyneuritic, tight-rope walker, robot, habit limping, choreic, knock-kneed, as on a sticky surface and as through water varieties. Understanding of these disorders has not made any progress over the last 70 years, except for the gradual delineation of new neuro-logical conditions designated as 'pseudohysterical' such as thalamic astasia, abasic gait apraxia and orthostatic tremor. Single case studies of hysterical motor disorder still warrant publication (Perez-Sales 1990).

The lack of progress in understanding these disorders is reflected in the lack of progress in treating them. Fishbain et al. (1988) list the following contem-porary treatments for conversion paralysis—physical therapy, occupational therapy, behaviour modification, vocational counselling, functional electrical stimulation and electromyogram feedback. A hundred years ago, Tourette (1895) listed the following treatments for hysteria—faradism, static electricity, magnetism, massage and hydrotherapy—and he commented that 'these treatment methods are not new'.

Like the psychiatric disorders in previous chapters, hysteria was considered neurologically during the second half of the last century, notably by Charcot and his school, with a further flurry of interest in a neurological interpretation of it in the wake of the encephalitis epidemic. At the Charcot centenary meeting of the Paris Neurological Society in 1925, Pienkowski (1925) reviewed Charcot's studies on the motor disorder of hysteria and drew attention to the value of these

for the study of normal and pathological motor function in man. He described
the following motor disorder as characteristic of hysteria:

> ...abnormal movements, which could be slow and sustained, often rhythmic or
> complex, affecting the head, trunk or limbs, bilaterally or unilaterally or sometimes
> only one extremity. The movements of the limbs were superimposed on an abnor-
> mality of posture fluctuating on a spectrum between the extremes of extension,
> adduction, internal rotation and carpo-pedal spasm on the one hand, and flexion,
> abduction, external rotation and characteristic posture of the extremities on the
> other. The effect was one of exaggerated associated movements, producing the effect
> of a balancing act, of a blacksmith, swimming, rowing, jumping or dancing. Muscles
> involved in respiration or chewing could be affected. Or there could be complex tics
> or co-ordinated movements such as crying, laughing, running or spinning with
> general excitability (Pienkowski 1925).

The closest neurological comparison was with encephalitis lethargica, where a
similar spectrum of abnormal movements could be found, which could be
provoked or abolished by suggestion and responded to psychotherapy (Salmon
1950).

This theme was explored by Radovici in a 1930 meeting of the Paris Neurological Society (Radovici 1930). With Marinesco and Dragenesco he had been one
of the first to describe oculogyric crisis as a post-encephalitic phenomenon in 1924
(Marinesco & Radovici 1926). When they had first observed the disorder they had
considered that it had a hysterical basis. It could be induced in affected patients
by strong emotion, suggestion, or seeing another affected patient when they had
never previously suffered from the condition ('mental contagion'). Attacks could
be aborted by persuasion or injections of distilled water, as well as anti-cholinergic
medication. He suggested that organic hysteroid states like post-encephalitic
oculogyric crisis could throw light on a possible pathophysiology of hysteria, just
as organic jacksonian epilepsy had on idiopathic epilepsy. The presentation by
Radovici at the meeting provoked a long discussion by the foremost French neurologists of the day—Souques, Roussy, Froment, Clovis Vincent and Babinski—who
were unanimous in squashing his suggestion of a possible neurological basis for
hysteria.

The English neurologist, Kinnier Wilson, however, thought differently. In
1931 (Wilson 1931), he wrote what is still the best modern paper on a neurological
approach to hysteria in his presidential address to the psychiatry section of the
Royal Society of Medicine. He felt that nothing was more typical in what he called
'the present era of psychological grace' than the comparative absence of research
of an objective and empirical kind on hysterical disorder. He favoured an
approach 'from below upwards', since he felt the gap between physiological and
psychological systems was scarcely likely to be bridged from the psychical side. He
analysed a series of motor disorders found in hysteria, suggesting a possible
cerebral basis for them by comparing them with motor disorder due to known
cerebral disorder.

One of these hysterical motor disorders was the phenomenon of 'defective inhibition of the antagonists' on elicited movement, described by his former chief Beevor in his 1904 Croonian lectures. For example, when a patient with an incomplete hysterical hemiplegia was asked to extend the elbow, the first muscle observed to contract was the supinator longus, an antagonist to the movement, followed immediately by triceps, succeeded by a confusion of to-and-fro movements due to alternate contraction of extensors and flexors of the elbow. Beevor had felt that this phenomenon was only found in hysterical paralysis and was pathognomonic of this condition. Wilson, however, had also demonstrated it in athetosis in his Croonian lectures of 1925. Here he had argued that the interference with the orderly innervation and de-innervation of prime movers and antagonists was produced by disordered function of cortical reflex arcs. He had also found the same phenomenon with lesions of the superior frontal cortex producing 'tonic innervation' and apraxias and now argued that the phenomenon found in both hysteria and certain neurological disorders could be due to the same neurophysiological dysfunction.

Another motor sign of hysteria was the shunting of innervation to other groups of muscles apart from the actual antagonists of the desired movement. When a patient with hysterical paresis of the arm was asked to grasp the examiner's fingers tightly, the patient gave the impression of great effort but the grasp remained weak while shoulder muscles and others equally distant from the long flexors contracted strongly. This 'shunting' sign was also found in some cases of muscle weakness due to structural lesions, although rarely so pronounced. Both these motor signs could be imitated by normal subjects, which some took as proof of simulation. Wilson found this argument superficial and worthless. It could equally be applied to accepted neurological conditions, such as polio, since complete muscle flaccidity and loss of tendon reflexes could be produced by a normal subject with practice. Wilson suggested that imitability might reflect the degree of cortical dysfunction in the impairment, but that the dysfunction of hysteria was just as genuine as any other, the hysteric patient being unable to inhibit antagonistic innervation or displacement of innervating stimuli.

Concerning abnormal movements, he could not accept that hysterical tremor, for example, considered physiologically, presented any separate or contrasting features to so-called organic tremors. The reputed differentiating features, such as variability, influence of psychic and emotional stimuli and dependence on the attention paid to it, he found demonstrably invalid. Organic tremors could sometimes fluctuate markedly, be irregular and be aggravated when the subject was observed. Hysterical tremors could sometimes be fixed and invariable. Differences between epileptic and hysterical fits were, he suggested, a matter of degree and not of kind. Clinical differences represented modifications in site and extent of cerebral affection, but not intrinsically or essentially different processes. He compared the opisthotonic and extensor pronation postures so commonly found in hysteria, illustrated in Richer's drawings of the 'arc de circle' phenomenon in Charcot's patients, with the decerebrate postures following organic mesencephalic transection, suggesting that only the mechanism of production was different (Wilson 1920). Hysterical paralysis could be associated with different disorders of tone ranging from rigidity and contracture to complete flaccidity. Cutaneous reflexes could be lost, typically the plantar and sometimes the abdominal response, usually in association with sensory loss. Ankle clonus could occur, as could urinary incontinence or retention.

Wilson felt 60 years ago that the progress of medical knowledge had been so gravely hampered by persistent use of the two terms 'organic' and 'functional' that it was high time they should be discarded for ever. The difference between hysterical and organic conditions was in the manner of the onset of the symptoms and the manner of their removal rather than in the symptoms themselves. His approach to hysteria was not typical for a twentieth-century neurologist. Much more typical is David Marsden's position (Marsden 1986) when, again to a psychiatric audience, he defined hysterical symptoms as complaints that are not fully explained by organic (visible) or 'true' functional (invisible but, perhaps, biochemical) neurological disease. Whilst honest, making ignorance about the cause of the disorder part of its definition does not encourage attempts to lessen this ignorance.

The validity of distinct hysterical signs and symptoms has seldom been subjected to even the most basic scientific analysis. Head, who wrote on the diagnosis of hysteria in the wake of World War I, based the diagnosis on the absence of a demonstrable organic clause and the presence of positive signs of hysteria. He admitted that much of the knowledge needed to distinguish these hysterical signs from those found in true neurological disorders was traditional and could not be found in textbooks. The first study of the validity of these signs was in fact by Gould et al. (1986). They took seven of the most accepted positive signs of hysteria—history of hypochondriasis, secondary gain, belle indifference, non-anatomical sensory loss, split of the mid-line by pain or vibration stimulation, changing boundaries of impaired sensation and give-way weakness—and examined 30 consecutive neurology admissions with acute structural brain disorder for these. All 30 had at least one of these seven features; 28 had two; 21 had three; 14 had four; five had five; two had six; and one had all seven features.

The second such study by Rolak (1988) confirmed the findings of the first. Two features commonly thought to indicate psychogenic sensory loss—exact splitting of the midline to pinprick and diminished vibratory sensation on the affected forehead—were examined in 100 consecutive patients complaining of hemifacial numbness, 80 of whom had organic lesions. Sensory loss split the midline in 20% of the non-organic and 7.5% of the organic patients. Vibration was unilaterally diminished in 95% of the non-organic and 86% of the organic patients. Thus the only two studies to date of classical signs of hysteria in neurological patients have completely invalidated their use in the diagnosis of 'non-neurological' disorder. Their time-honoured use for this purpose had more to do with the re-inforcement of artificial distinctions between neurological and psychiatric disorder than the spirit of scientific enquiry.

The validity of a diagnosis of hysteria has repeatedly been called into question, for example, after the famous follow-up study of patients with a diagnosis of hysteria made at the National Hospital, Queen Square (Slater 1965) showing that a significant proportion had neurological disorder, which could not be diagnosed at the time of their initial presentation. Paradoxically, this may have had the effect of discouraging a renewed interest in the neurological aspects of hysterical disorder, as has occurred over the last 25 years for other psychiatric disorders but which for hysteria remains long overdue.

MENTAL HANDICAP

Motor disorder forms a significant part of the many disabilities of patients with mental handicap, and especially of those with severe handicap. This has been recognised since the first descriptions of motor disorder in the mentally handicapped at the beginning of this century, but the interpretation put on the motor disorder, as for psychiatric disorder generally over this period, has varied considerably. The early literature is well reviewed by Vermeylen (1923) and Earl (1934). Opinion was divided at the beginning of this century, some regarding the motor disorders of severe mental handicap as the normal catatoniform movements of certain periods in child development, others as similar to the catatonic disorders associated with psychotic illness recently described by Kahlbaum. Accepting them as genuinely catatonic created problems as the majority of subjects with severe mental handicap would have had to be diagnosed as having dementia praecox. Celles de Naudascher in 1908, in a study of 278 mentally handicapped children and adults, and 230 non-handicapped controls had found significant motor impairment in 75% of 'idiots' (severe mental handicap), 44% of 'imbeciles' (moderate mental handicap), 24% of 'feeble-minded' (mild mental handicap) and only 2% of non-handicapped children.

Vermeylen studied 127 mentally handicapped boys aged between 8 and 20 years, whose degree of mental handicap was established by the new Binet–Simon tests. He performed a clinical examination of motor function including tendon and cutaneous reflexes, tone, persistence of postures, motor power, manual dexterity, synkinesis, gait and speech, respiratory and sphincter function. He found that motor disorder was very common in his subjects and that there was a greater prevalence in those with more severe levels of handicap. Earl felt that motor abnormalities occurred in practically all patients with severe mental handicap. He studied 135 such patients and described various catatonic signs including catalepsy, echolalia, echopraxia, disorder of tone, flexion postures such as bowing of the head or the 'intra-uterine' position, mutism, negativism and repetitive, rhythmical and semi-purposeful movements, as well as sudden outbursts of violent impulsive movement. In 38 of the 135 patients, the disorder was so prominent that he named it the primitive catatonic psychosis of idiocy. He considered this motor disorder as identical to that found in patients with schizophrenia and argued against the psycho-analytic interpretations of motor disorder, which were being suggested at this time in both schizophrenia and mental handicap.

As in psychiatry generally at this time, a psychological explanatory paradigm then became the prevalent one in the field of mental handicap. O'Gorman (1979), for example, felt that, although organic factors had to be postulated to explain the increased liability to motor abnormalities of the severely handicapped, psychogenic rather than physical causes were responsible for the vast majority of motor abnormalities in mental handicap. He described mannerisms, motor habits and stereotypies as serving a useful purpose, fulfilling a defensive role in a vulnerable individual. As in psychiatry generally, a psychological paradigm had the effect of reducing interest in motor disorder. Compared to the detailed description of this motor disorder earlier in the century, motor disorders in mental handicap were dealt with very simply. Abnormal movements in the mentally handicapped were often all lumped together as 'self-stimulation' with no attempt to study their prevalence (Kalachnik 1984), in marked contrast to studies of abnormal movements attributed to neuroleptic medication in mentally handicapped patients after this was introduced.

As in psychiatry generally, an arbitrary distinction between neurological and psychiatric motor disorder makes estimates of total prevalence of motor disorder problematic. With colleagues, I examined the motor disorders of 236 in-patients in one hospital for the mentally handicapped (Rogers et al. 1991), not making any a priori distinction between neurological and psychiatric motor disorder.

The following disorders were found:

- *Abnormality of posture* (70%): flexion of the head when they were lying on their bed with no pillow, 48%; head flexion when upright, 19%; marked dorsal kyphosis, 13%; arm flexion, 24%; finger flexion, 12%; hyperpronation/ abduction/hyperextension postures of the arms or trunk, 14%; persistence of postures, 4%.
- *Disorder of tone* (52%): increased tone in the neck, 26%; increased tone in the arms, 25%; decreased tone in the neck, 15%; decreased tone in the arms, 11%; spasticity, 9%; gegenhalten, 6%; cogwheeling, 1%.
- *Disorder of purposive movement* (98%): generally underactive, 18%; needing help or encouragement with washing and dressing, 54%; and with eating, 16%; slowness, freezing or abruptness of movement, 23%; paresis of one or more limbs, 10%. On request: not performing independent finger movements, 86%; not performing arm movements, 39%; not performing whole body movements, 7%; 40% showed echopraxia.
- *Disorder of activity* (62%): general overactivity, 15%; behavioural outbursts with shouting and swearing, threatening behaviour or actual assaults on others, 43%; objectional habits such as smearing faeces, 18%; destructive, 16%; 'delinquent', 14%; a history of self-injury, 15%.
- *Abnormal movements of the head, trunk or limbs* (44%): brief and random,

7%; semi-purposeful, 24%; rhythmic, 11%; sustained and spasmodic, 4%; tremor, 4%; showed complex or simple tics, 12%. One patient had myoclonic jerking.

- *Abnormality of gait* (68%): gait slow, 24%; shuffling, 28%; no associated movements, 38%; exaggerated associated movements, 3%; spastic gait, 6%; ataxic gait, 1%; needing a walking aid, 5%; able only to crawl, 3%; confined to a wheelchair, 5%.

- *Abnormal spontaneous eye movements* (38%): roving semi-purposeful movements, 26%; abrupt conjugate deviation of the eyes, 13%; 'to-and-fro' movements, 2%; no eye contact with the examiner, 9%; staring, 3%.

- *Obvious abnormality of blinking* (18%): increased blinking, 9%; decreased blinking, 6%; rapid bursts of blinking, 4%.

- *Abnormal facial movements or posture* (63%): spasmodic contractions of one or more facial muscles, 27%; fluid random movements, mainly round the mouth, 28%; lack of facial expression, 17%; rhythmic movements, tremor or tics of the oro-facial muscles, 8%.

- *Abnormality of speech production* (89%): totally mute, 8%; partially mute, 42%; dysarthria, 36%; unintelligible speech, 46%; impaired volume, timbre or rate of intelligible speech, 15%; stuttering or palilalia, 4%; echolalia, 6%.

The study was modelled on that which I had previously carried out on 100 patients with severe psychiatric illness, most with a case-note diagnosis of schizophrenia (Rogers 1985). Table 5·1 shows the % patients with at least one abnormality in each of the 10 categories of motor disorder in both studies.

Table 5.1 Percentage of patients with at least one abnormality in each of 10 categories of motor disorder in two studies

	Patients with mental handicap (%) ($n = 236$)	Patients with severe schizophrenic illness (%) ($n = 100$)
Posture	70	86
Tone	52	85
Purposive movement	98	97
Activity	62	64
Abnormal movements of head, trunk or limbs	44	67
Gait	68	48
Abnormal eye movements	38	48
Blinking	18	38
Abnormal facial movements	63	74
Speech production	89	95
Abnormality in:		
At least one category	100	100
At least five categories	73	91

The ages of the mentally handicapped patients ranged from 24 to 82 years and they had been patients in the hospital for between 1 and 69 years. There was no association between the amount of motor disorder and age or length of admission, thus age-related cerebral changes or institutionalisation did not significantly contribute to the amount of motor disorder. In 35%, some idea of the aetiology of the mental handicap was known; 76% had associated physical disorder, past or present; 55% had abnormalities of tendon reflexes, plantar response, pupils, squint or nystagmus; 60% were taking non-neuroleptic medication. The amount of motor disorder was not related to any of these parameters.

The severity of mental handicap was mild in 15%, moderate in 22%, severe in 23% and profound in 42%; 44% had associated psychiatric disorder, mostly behaviour disorder; 27% had a history of epilepsy; 32% were currently receiving neuroleptic medication, a further 26% had received such medication in the past and 42% had never received any. There was a significant correlation between the amount of motor disorder and the severity of mental handicap, the presence of associated psychiatric disorder, the presence of epilepsy and the use of neuroleptic medication either currently or previously. As in the study of severe psychiatric illness, neuroleptic medication was neither necessary nor sufficient to produce any of the motor disorders.

6 Motor Disorder and Medication

NEUROLEPTIC MEDICATION

The issue of the role of medication in motor disorder in psychiatry first became a major one after the introduction of neuroleptic medication in the 1950s. This produced a wide spectrum of extrapyramidal disorder, including parkinsonism, akathisia, dyskinesia and dystonia.

Treatment of psychiatric patients with chlorpromazine was first reported by French authors in 1952, followed by reports of treatment with reserpine. Extrapyramidal disorder due to the treatment was first reported by Swiss authors in 1953. At a meeting of the Societe Medico-psychologique in Paris in 1954, Hans Steck (1954) from Lausanne reported a reversible, dose-related extrapyramidal syndrome, including parkinsonism and akathisia, in 111 of 299 patients, most with a diagnosis of chronic schizophrenia, treated with chlorpromazine or reserpine.

Steck did not confine himself to clinical description but discussed the theoretical implications of his findings. He compared the effect of the medication to that of encephalitis lethargica with which he was well acquainted. The initial sedation produced by the drug corresponded to the lethargic phase of the encephalitis. This was followed in about 40% of cases by a parkinsonian syndrome, as following the encephalitis. The drug-induced disorder, however, evolved more rapidly, like a speeded up film.

Steck recalled cases of patients with chronic schizophrenia who had been affected by encephalitis lethargica and in whom this had produced a beneficial effect on their psychosis as they developed a parkinsonian syndrome. This beneficial effect of encephalitis superadded to schizophrenia had also been mentioned by his colleague Professor Staehelin at a conference in Switzerland the year before. Where Staehelin had proposed a theory of antagonism between schizophrenia and encephalitis to explain this effect, Steck suggested that the encephalitis and the new medication acted by speeding up the natural history of certain psychotic illnesses, which typically progressed from an initial phase of acute agitation with overactivity to one of akinetic underactivity and then sometimes even spontaneous cure. He thus suggested a theory of interaction between drug and disease induced motor disorder: this could be called the 'Steck hypothesis'.

Steck also suggested that since encephalitis lethargica had been shown to produce most of its effects on the upper brainstem and extrapyramidal motor system, the new medication acted on the same brain systems. His theory of interaction between drug and disease effects would thus support disorder of the same brain systems in psychotic patients, as he had suggested some 30 years before in his study of the extrapyramidal disorder associated with psychiatric illness (Steck 1926, 1927).

Most of his audience at the 1954 meeting, however, were sceptical of the drug-induced extrapyramidal syndrome he was describing. French authors were at this time using smaller doses of chlorpromazine than the Swiss. Pierre Deniker, who was in the audience, said that he had never seen an extrapyramidal syndrome follow the use of chlorpromazine in the doses they were currently using for schizophrenia and suggested that Steck was describing a modification of catatonic disorder of tone.

In the same year, 1954, Haase (1958, 1961) reported from Germany on the effects of chlorpromazine and reserpine on the size of handwriting, which could be used to monitor treatment with these drugs. He too felt these effects were extrapyramidal and could be compared to a speeded-up version ('tempo cinematographique accelere') of the effects of encephalitis lethargica. He found that the therapeutic effects of the new drugs were necessarily associated with the production of a mild, but not severe, akinesia. Again he describes this idea as having met initial scepticism.

Within a year of Steck's and Haase's papers, however, the production of extrapyramidal symptoms by chlorpromazine and reserpine had been accepted, and Delay and Deniker (1956) proposed the term 'neuroleptic' for these drugs because of their neurological effects, and like Steck and Haase, considered these effects as central to the drugs' mode of action.

Some felt there was no necessary relationship between the neurological effects of the medication and its therapeutic action. Brooks (1956), for example, reported the treatment over 16 months of 386 psychotic patients with chlorpromazine and reserpine. The initial sign of improvement in the psychotic disorder often coincided with the onset of obvious extrapyramidal disorder but the patient's progress was enhanced when extrapyramidal dysfunction was relieved. Others felt there had to be a link between neurological and therapeutic effect. Freyhan (1957) reported the treatment over 2 years of 653 patients with chlorpromazine and reserpine. He felt that this experience supported his initial impression that an extrapyramidal syndrome was a regular effect of neuroleptic drugs and part and parcel of their therapeutic action, and that it was arbitrary to define borderlines between therapeutic hypomotility and early signs of parkinsonism. Kruse (1957) compared the therapeutic effect of neuroleptic drugs to the mental symptoms— bradyphrenia and emotional indifference—of parkinsonism and felt that the therapeutic action of these drugs illustrated the close relationship between schizophrenia and the extrapyramidal system. Denham and Carrick (1959–60) reported a clinical trial of a new phenothiazine in 40 schizophrenic patients showing a definite relationship between the therapeutic efficacy and the extrapyramidal disturbance produced by the drug.

A major symposium on the extrapyramidal effects of neuroleptic medication was held in Montreal in 1960 (Symposium 1960). The question of the relationship of these extrapyramidal effects and therapeutic efficacy was debated at length. Everyone agreed that neuroleptic medication was characterised by its neurological effects but opinion was divided on whether these were responsible for the drugs' therapeutic effector or were merely side-effects. Delay and Deniker (1960) felt that these two points of view were not in fact incompatible. The intensity of neurological effects produced by particular neuroleptics was by and large related to their therapeutic potential but some of these neurological effects could be relieved without diminishing their therapeutic activity. If the neurological effects were not regarded as a unitary phenomenon then certain motor effects might be essential and others superfluous.

At the time the conference took place in 1960, the psychological paradigm was still the dominant one in psychiatry. The conference proceedings included attempts to explain the mode of action of these new psychotropic agents from the standpoint of this paradigm. 'Introjective mechanisms', by which the 'good physician was orally incorporated in the form of a pill', and the . . . 'intrapsychic meaning of side-effects' were discussed and Freud reverentially quoted:

> the future may teach us how to exercise a direct influence by means of particular chemical substances upon the amount of energy and their distributions in the apparatus of the mind (Freud, quoted in Azima & Sarwer-Foner 1960).

Akathisia, or subjective and objective motor restlessness, as a result of neuroleptic medication was again first described by Steck in his 1954 paper. It occupied the middle ground between neurology and psychiatry. The term had been introduced by Haskovec (1901) to describe the spontaneously occurring disorder in two cases—one of hysteria and one of neurasthenia—where he suggested it represented functional sub-cortical overactivity. It was later described as part of post-encephalitic parkinsonism. In neurological textbooks such as Wilson's (1940), it appeared both in the chapter on parkinsonism and the chapter on psychoneuroses. Wilson considered it a hysterical phenomenon. Winkelman, discussing akathisia in the 1960 conference on neuroleptic medication (Winkelman 1960), described neurophysiological and psychological explanations of akathisia as different ways of talking about the same thing.

By the time the 1960 conference took place, 23 different phenothiazine derivatives had been assessed. Extrapyramidal side-effects continued to be a feature of later drugs introduced for the treatment of psychotic disorders. In 1965, Bishop et al. (1965) reviewed the few published controlled studies of a possible relationship between therapeutic response and extrapyramidal side-effects. None of these, except one which they felt lacked methodological sophistication, supported such a relationship. They performed their own controlled studies and concluded that gross extrapyramidal side-effects bore no direct relationship to drug response but that the possibility of a relationship between clinical improvement and subclinical extrapyramidal system disturbance had not been excluded. They described this possibility as intriguing and possibly shedding light on the neurophysiological correlates of psychotic disorder. Some later studies supported the suggestion of a relationship of clinical improvement with mild but not severe extrapyramidal disorder (Simpson & Kunz-Bartholini 1968), but this avenue was not further explored. A new drug-induced motor disorder—tardive dyskinesia—took centre stage.

TARDIVE DYSKINESIA

Schonecker (1957) described persistent smacking movements of the lips and licking of the lips developing in three patients after a few days to 8 weeks of treatment with chlorpromazine and reserpine. The three patients had a diagnosis of cerebral sclerosis with depression or anxiety. Two years later, Sigwald et al. (1959b) reported four cases of persistent oro-facial dyskinesia starting 3–18 months after continuous treatment with neuroleptic medication for pain syndromes, anxiety and obsessional neurosis. These are considered to be the first two reports of what came to be called 'tardive dyskinesia', a term coined by Faurbye in 1964. Most of the subsequently reported cases were in patients with chronic schizophrenia.

From the outset, there was difficulty distinguishing the movements in such patients from motor features of their illness, which had never been the subject of intensive study. When the findings of one of the first studies were presented (Hunter et al. 1964), they met scepticism because the movements being described were felt to be those of chronic psychiatric illness (Earl 1983). Studies which included untreated as well as treated patients showed that neuroleptic medication was not a necessary cause of the disorder. Brandon et al. (1971) examined all the residents of a regional mental hospital who had been there more than 3 months, for the presence of oro-facial dyskinesia. The patients had a wide variety of diagnoses. Oro-facial dyskinesia was present in 22% of the 491 currently receiving neuroleptic medication, 36% of the 134 who had received such medication previously and 20% of the 285 who had never received any or if they had for under 3 months.

By 1967, 600 cases of tardive dyskinesia had been reported in 37 papers and by 1972, 1800 cases in 97 papers (Crane 1973). Despite the number of studies, facts concerning tardive dyskinesia were difficult to establish. There was an increased prevalence and severity with advancing age, but little consistent association with length or intensity of treatment with neuroleptics. There was no consensus on how the abnormal movements were best classified. Different investigators at the same symposium, for example, could characterise them as choreiform (Klawans 1983) or stereotypic (Fahn 1983). Some remained sceptical of neuroleptic medication being a necessary and sufficient cause of the syndrome (Curran 1973; Turek 1975; Turner 1988), but most investigators adopted the view that neuroleptic medication was the main cause. The term came to include any hyperkinesia found in patients on long-term neuroleptic medication and the concept was extended to other abnormal movements or clinical disorder described as tardive dystonia, tardive oculogyric crisis, tardive tourettism, tardive akathisia, and tardive dementia.

The symptoms of tardive dyskinesia can be improved or suppressed by neuroleptic medication in about two-thirds of patients (Jeste & Wyatt 1982), just as choreiform (parakinetic) movements in untreated schizophrenic patients could be improved by neuroleptic medication (Fish 1964). The disorder persists after discontinuing neuroleptic medication. Glazer et al. (1990) studied 49 chronic psychiatric patients for a mean of 40 weeks after the discontinuation of neuroleptic medication. Complete and persistent reversibility of tardive dyskinesia occurred in only one patient. The course of the movement disorder following discontinuation of the medication appeared to be related to the type and history of psychiatric illness. Non-schizophrenic patients, the majority of whom had affective disorder, were over three times more likely to show improvement of the movements than were patients with schizophrenia. Permanent neuroleptic-induced tardive dyskinesia, however, has been reported in individuals without previous neurological or severe psychiatric disorder (Sigwald et al. 1959b; Klawans et al. 1974).

Longitudinal investigations of tardive dyskinesia in the same patients have shown that the disorder can fluctuate even on a steady dose of neuroleptic medication. Robinson and McCreadie (1986) measured the prevalence of tardive dyskinesia in schizophrenic patients from a discrete geographical area in 1981, 1982 and 1984. The prevalence at these three times was 31%, 27% and 30%, respectively, but in only 12% of patients was dyskinesia present at all three assessments. Bergen et al. (1989) carried out five consecutive annual examinations using the Abnormal Involuntary Movement Scale (AIMS) on 101 chronic psychiatric patients on long-term neuroleptics. At each examination, the prevalence of patients, using a criterion score on the AIMS, in the whole group with tardive dyskinesia remained constant at around 66%, but the individual patients making up this positive percentage each time differed.

The longest follow-up studies to date have shown conflicting results. Koshino et al. (1991) followed 28 patients with tardive dyskinesia for up to 12 years while they remained on neuroleptic medication. Abnormal movements did not disappear in any patient but could worsen, improve, remain the same or fluctuate in severity over the period of observation. McClelland et al. (1991) performed a follow-up study after 16 years on 99 survivors of the 910 mental hospital population originally surveyed by the same group (Brandon et al. 1971). The patients followed up had non-organic brain syndromes, mostly schizophrenia. The prevalence of dyskinesia in these patients rose from 18.4% to 46.5% over this period, and this increase was associated with neuroleptic dosage.

Steck's hypothesis that neuroleptic medication made motor disorder appear earlier than it would have in the natural history of the disorder being treated was never tested. This is now more difficult because control groups of patients never exposed to neuroleptic medication are difficult to find, but the few studies with matched control groups of treated and untreated patients at different stages of their illnesses would seem to support his hypothesis. Chorfi & Moussaoui (1985) were able to assess 50 patients in Morocco who had had a schizophrenic illness for under 12 months and who had never received any neuroleptic medication. They examined them for the abnormal movements of tardive dyskinesia, using the standardised Abnormal Involuntary Movement Scale (AIMS) rating scale, and compared this to the same examination of 50 age- and sex-matched patients at a similar stage of their schizophrenic illness who had received neuroleptic medication, and 50 age-matched controls: seven (14%) of the 50 treated, one (2%) of the 50 never-treated patients and none of the controls showed abnormal movements. At this stage of the patients' schizophrenic illness, neuroleptic medication seemed definitely associated with the apparition of abnormal movements.

Owens et al. (1982) were able to study a group of patients at a much later stage of their severe chronic schizophrenic illnesses who had never been treated with neuroleptic medication because of the 'anti-psychiatry' philosophy of the consultant who had cared for them. They compared 47 such patients with 364 similar patients who had received neuroleptic medication, using two standardised rating scales including the AIMS. Movements considered to be 'stereotypic' or 'manneristic' were not rated for assessment with one scale, but otherwise no a priori judgements were made concerning the source of the movement disorders. The patients' medication history was only checked after their examination. There was no statistically significant difference in ratings for abnormal movements between treated patients and those never treated with neuroleptic medication using either scale but, when age was taken into account, the increased prevalence of abnormal movements in treated patients became more pronounced (Crow et al. 1982). Using the same criterion of severity on the AIMS as did Chorfi and Moussaoui in their study of more acute patients, 70% of the 364 neuroleptic-treated and 53% of the 47 never-treated patients showed abnormal movements. At this late stage of their schizophrenic illnesses, then, the influence of medication, although still apparent, was much less pronounced than in the early stages of the illness, as shown in Chorfi and Moussaoui's study, thus supporting the Steck hypothesis.

In their discussion of their results, the authors suspected that their finding, that spontaneous involuntary movement disorder with a predominantly oro-facial distribution could be a feature of severe chronic schizophrenia even when the illness was unmodified by neuroleptic drugs, might be considered heretical. Initial reaction to their findings suggested just this. The findings, however, were supported by other studies of untreated patients with chronic schizophrenia, although these were naturally difficult to find. In their survey of all known schizophrenic patients from a discrete geographical area (McCreadie et al. 1982), a prevalence of tardive dyskinesia of 31% was found. This included two (29%) of the seven patients with no record of ever having received neuroleptic medication. In my study of 100 patients with severe psychiatric illness (Rogers 1985), most of whom had a case-note diagnosis of schizophrenia, altogether 35% had fluid, random peri-oral movements. This included three (38%) of the eight patients with no record of ever having received neuroleptic medication. During their studies of tardive dyskinesia in schizophrenia, Waddington and Youssef (1990) came across four schizophrenic patients in their ninth or tenth decade who had never been treated with neuroleptics, with involuntary oro-facial movements indistinguishable from tardive dyskinesia.

One patient group where reliable untreated control groups are much more readily available is that of mental handicap. Interestingly, this obvious field for controlled studies was hardly exploited until recently. Kalachnik (1984) reviewed four different studies from 1975 to 1982 of tardive dyskinesia in mentally handicapped subjects, which had examined a total of 225 subjects all treated with neuroleptic medication: he reported an average prevalence of tardive dyskinesia of 29%. In a further study of tardive dyskinesia in the mentally handicapped, Richardson et al. (1986) examined the 299 of 721 residents in an institution for the retarded who had received neuroleptics for at least one year in the previous five and found a prevalence of tardive dyskinesia of 30%. The underlying assumption of all these studies was that neuroleptic medication was entirely responsible for the motor disorder being described. None included a control group of untreated patients. Nevertheless, Richardson and colleagues used the prevalence of dyskinesia found in their study, which was similar to the prevalence found by the Northwick Park group in untreated schizophrenic patients (Owens et al. 1982), to question the apparent lack of exposure to neuroleptic medication of the patients in the Northwick Park study.

More recent studies have included control groups. Stone et al. (1988) studied the entire population of 1282 residents in a large hospital for the developmentally handicapped: 55% had been treated with anti-psychotic drugs at some stage and 45% had no history of such treatment. Dyskinesia was present in 48% of the treated group and 48% of the non-treated group. In our study (Rogers et al. 1991) of the motor disorder of 236 in-patients in one hospital for the mentally handicapped, 76 patients were currently receiving neuroleptic medication, 61 had previously but were not currently receiving such medication and 99 had no record of ever having received any. Motor assessments were performed blind to treatment status. Every motor abnormality found was present in untreated as well as treated individuals. Neuroleptic medication appeared to modify the expression of the motor disorder rather than producing it de nova. For example, in the 76 patients currently receiving neuroleptic medication, the prevalence of 'fluid, random perioral movements', the core feature of tardive dyskinesia, was 34%. The prevalence of the same movements in the 61 patients who had previously received neuroleptic medication was 20%, and in the 99 who had apparently never received any, 27%.

An excellent literature review and critique of tardive dyskinesia has been provided by Waddington (1989). According to him:

> Tardive dyskinesia is one of the few topics of scientific enquiry concerning which studies are entertained when they fail to include features that would be deemed mandatory in virtually all other areas of neuroscience research (Waddington 1989).

Methodological problems have permeated every aspect of the syndrome. Standardised rating scales used to measure tardive dyskinesia can only assess involuntary movements. They are not diagnostic instruments and cannot differentiate the involuntary movements of tardive dyskinesia from other involuntary movements. Normal subjects are not a valid control group for patient populations since they fail to control for the factor of the disease process that resulted in their requirement for treatment.

Waddington summarises the available literature as follows:

- Involuntary movements indistinguishable from those of tardive dyskinesia are exceptionally rare in the normal elderly, free of medical or neuropsychiatric disorders and without exposure to neuroleptics, even up to the tenth decade of life. The prevalence of such movements in 1032 such subjects assessed in five different studies was 1.3%.

- Inclusion of medical disorders in such populations is associated with an increased prevalence of abnormal movements similar to tardive dyskinesia, even in the absence of neuropsychiatric disorders and exposure to neuroleptics. The prevalence of these movements in 1584 such subjects in six different studies was 8.2%.

- Involuntary movements, particularly those of the orofacial region, which typify tardive dyskinesia, can be seen to an appreciable extent in patient populations with major psychosis or neurodegenerative and neurodevelopmental disorders that have not been exposed to neuroleptics. The prevalence of such movements in 2372 such subjects in 12 different studies was 23.4%.

- Considering eight studies where the same assessment procedure was applied to treated and untreated, though not necessarily matched, groups within different neuropsychiatric populations, the prevalence of abnormal movements in 1788 untreated subjects was 29.6% and in 1854 treated subjects 41.2% (Waddington 1989).

For Waddington, a parsimonious conclusion from this analysis is that the prevalence of involuntary movements in untreated neuropsychiatric disorders appears to have been underestimated and that long-term treatment with neuroleptic drugs makes it more likely that such movements will emerge rather than creating them de novo. He concludes that the available evidence supports the view that long-term treatment with neuroleptics does not 'cause' tardive dyskinesia but rather interacts with a neurological process that is an intrinsic component of the disorder being treated, hastening the emergence of a buccal–lingual–masticatory motor disorder that has a high likelihood of ultimately occurring spontaneously with increasing cerebral dysfunction. The 'Steck hypothesis' thus seems vindicated.

OVERLAP OF DRUG-INDUCED MOTOR DISORDER AND PSYCHIATRIC DISORDER

A close relationship between drug-induced motor disorder and psychiatric disorder has been noted from the outset. Deniker (1960), for example, described how acute dystonic reactions due to neuroleptic medication were first described as 'hysterical' or 'hysteria-like', much as had been the case when similar symptoms were first noted after encephalitis lethargica. Like these dystonic 'crises' following the encephalitis, neuroleptic-induced dystonic episodes could be precipitated by emotional stress or the sight of other patients with similar attacks, and suppressed temporarily by suggestion. Deniker also described the exacerbation of catatonic states and the appearance of catatonic symptoms in schizophrenic patients who had not shown them before with neuroleptic medication.

The parkinsonism seen in patients treated with neuroleptic medication is rare in experimental animals treated with the same medication, where catalepsy or catatonia was produced. Already in 1959, Sigwald et al. (1959a) had suggested that catatonia and parkinsonism represented different severity of the same motor disorder. Catatonia precipitated by neuroleptic medication in patients with schizophrenia, mania, borderline personality, obsessive–compulsive disorder or drug abuse with no previous history of psychiatric disorder or treatment with neuroleptic medication, as well as exacerbation of catatonia in catatonic schizophrenia, has been repeatedly reported (May 1959; Williams 1972; De 1973; Gelenberg & Mandel 1977; Weinberger & Kelly 1977; Brenner & Rheuban 1978; Hoffman 1986). These catatonic symptoms could be accompanied by parkinsonian features and both catatonic and parkinsonian symptoms responded to withdrawal of the neuroleptic or the addition of anti-parkinsonian medication. It was suggested that there was a spectrum of severity of extrapyramidal disorder produced by neuroleptic medication ranging from acute dystonias and dyskinesias, akathisia and parkinsonism to catatonia and the neuroleptic malignant syndrome, with these last representing the most severe extrapyramidal effect.

The most severe form of catatonia can be fatal. In the pre-neuroleptic era it was called 'lethal catatonia'. The neuroleptic malignant syndrome (Kellam 1990) is a neuroleptic-induced iatrogenic form, but can also be produced by other drugs altering dopamine function. It consists of severe akinesia, rigidity, catalepsy and hyperthermia with autonomic dysfunction, peak temperature being closely associated with survival. It can occur with any of the conditions, physical or psychiatric, associated with catatonia and the particular associated diagnosis does not affect the outcome. It can present with an acute catatonic state and no previous history of psychiatric disorder (White & Robins 1991). This supports the view that catatonia and the neuroleptic malignant syndrome share a common neurochemical basis (Fricchione 1985).

Neuroleptic medication can also exacerbate other features of psychotic illness, including excitability, restlessness, over-talkativeness, anxiety, fearfulness, aggressiveness, withdrawal, somatic delusions, paranoid delusions, auditory hallucinations, thought disorder and suicidal preoccupation (Curry 1971; van Putten et al. 1974; Barnes & Bridges 1980). In their systematic study of 80 patients with schizophrenia, van Putten and colleagues found evidence of such exacerbation in nine patients. They felt that this exacerbation of psychosis could be viewed as an extrapyramidal equivalent since it occurred with phenothiazines associated with a high incidence of extrapyramidal side-effects, was dose-related, was always associated with recognised extrapyramidal disorder (mainly akathisia), was similar to mental symptoms reported in extrapyramidal disorders such as Parkinson's disease, and was dramatically reversed by anti-parkinsonian agents.

The abnormal movements of tardive dyskinesia can be strongly associated with psychotic symptomatology in the same patients. Degkwitz (1969) carried out a study under double blind conditions where the neuroleptic medication of 53 of 87 patients with chronic schizophrenia, who had been taking them for at least two years, was abruptly stopped: 15 patients developed hyperkinesias for the first time and 10 patients, who already had hyperkinesias, showed worsening of these. All of these 25 patients also showed worsening of their psychotic symptoms, whereas there was no change in mental state in any of the patients who did not develop abnormal movements or the intensification of previous abnormal movements. Nadel (1978) reported the appearance of abnormal movements indistinguishable from tardive dyskinesia in two patients with schizophrenia on steady doses of neuroleptic medication following severe psychosocial stresses. These movements lasted for periods of 2 weeks and 2 months, respectively, and were associated with transient severe exacerbation of their psychiatric symptoms. The abnormal movements and abnormal mental state improved together.

Waddington et al. (1987) have studied the association of the abnormal movements of tardive dyskinesia with 22 different variables in 88 chronic schizophrenic in-patients. The presence and severity of oro-facial dyskinesia was strongly and consistently associated with the presence of marked cognitive dysfunction and muteness, in notable contrast to the paucity of associations with indexes of prior treatment with neuroleptics. When they studied 40 out-patients with bipolar affective disorder and exposure to neuroleptics and lithium (Waddington et al. 1989), they made similar findings. The primary association with the presence and severity of abnormal movements was again cognitive impairment and features of their illness, rather than the neuroleptic or other medication prescribed. They suggested that some neurological process in bipolar affective disorder, as well as schizophrenia, could be an important vulnerability factor for the emergence of involuntary movements during long-term neuroleptic treatment. These findings have been supported by those of Manschreck et al. (1990) who examined abnormal movements, cognitive impairment, psychopathology and medication history in 22 patients with chronic schizophrenia. Those with involuntary movements had more negative symptomatology, greater impairment on voluntary motor tasks, lower pre-morbid intelligence and a trend to poorer current cognitive ability. They did not differ in age, length of illness and medication variables from those without such movements. They suggested that 'abnormal involuntary movements' was a more precise term than tardive dyskinesia.

'Tardive' abnormal movements can be associated with different phases of the psychiatric disorder being treated. In bipolar affective disorder, tardive dyskinesia or tardive dystonia can be most pronounced in the depressive phase disappearing completely or almost completely during the manic phase (Cutler et al. 1981; Potter et al. 1983; Lal et al. 1988; Sachdev 1989; Yazici et al. 1991) or, conversely, subside or disappear completely during the depressive phase (Keshavan & Goswany 1983; Bhugra & Baker 1990). Jawed and Singh (1989) reported the case of a 50-year-old borderline mentally handicapped person with a 26-year history of schizophrenia and continuous treatment with neuroleptic medication, who had recurrent psychotic episodes with delusions and agitation. For the last 5 years, these episodes had been associated with tardive dyskinesia. Over a 4-year period he had 19 psychotic episodes. With each episode he developed the florid features of tardive dyskinesia, which disappeared with the remission of the psychotic symptoms, even though he remained on the same doses of neuroleptic medication. The association of abnormal movements with particular phases of a psychiatric illness was recognised before the introduction of neuroleptic medication. Bleuler (1923, p. 406) described dystonic pursing of the lips or 'snout cramp' accompanying melancholic phases and disappearing during manic phases in a patient with schizophrenia.

Relatively little study has been made of how easy it is to distinguish drug-induced extrapyramidal and psychiatric motor disorder. Weiden et al. (1987) compared clinicians' recognition of the major extrapyramidal syndromes in 48 of 58 consecutive admissions to a psychiatric in-patient clinic with independent blind diagnoses by clinical researchers using standardised ratings. They found that akinesia could be diagnosed clinically as depression, akathisia as agitation, restlessness as 'acting out', and acute dystonic reactions as 'psychotic behaviour'; these last could be considered 'hysteric' by nursing staff. Meisalas et al. (1989) showed videotapes of autistic children with stereotypies or neuroleptic-related dyskinesias to three experienced raters, who were 'blind' to the children's medication status or history. Of the 16 with stereotypies who had never been exposed to neuroleptic medication, one-third to one-half were diagnosed as showing tardive dyskinesia. Of the four with withdrawal dyskinesia from neuroleptic medication, one-quarter to three-quarters were diagnosed as showing non-drug related stereotypies. Further similar studies in different patient groups would be a fruitful area to explore.

THE 'CONFLICT OF PARADIGMS' HYPOTHESIS

This states (Rogers 1985) that a rigid division of motor disorder into catatonic or extrapyramidal is not possible. For historical reasons 'catatonic' has been regarded as psychiatric and 'extrapyramidal' as neurological. Motor disorder in patients with psychiatric illness, such as schizophrenia, is regarded as 'catatonic'if it is felt to be due to their underlying disease process and 'extrapyramidal' if it is felt to be due to exposure to neuroleptic medication. The orthodox view would be that distinguishing between these two is quite straightforward if care is taken to eliminate confounding motor disorder in the middle range of the spectrum of motor disorder found in such patients, which is not clearly disease- or medication-based. The 'conflict of paradigms' hypothesis predicts that an absolute distinction between catatonic disease-based and extrapyramidal treatment-based motor disorder is impossible however hard one tries. McKenna et al. (1991) have recently put this to the test by deliberately setting out to distinguish 'catatonic' and 'extrapyramidal' motor disorder present in the same patients.

Altogether, 93 patients meeting recognised criteria for schizophrenia were examined. They comprised acute, rehabilitation and long-stay hospitalised patients in approximately equal numbers. Catatonic motor disorder was assessed using the catatonic items from the Modified Rogers Scale (Lund et al. 1991) and the Behavioural Observation Schedule (Atakan & Cooper 1989). Extrapyramidal motor disorder was assessed using scales for parkinsonism and tardive dyskinesia (Webster 1968; Simpson & Angus 1970; Simpson et al. 1979). The motor disorder of 75 of the patients was assessed by two examiners simultaneously but independently, and that of 40 patients by two examiners on separate occasions on the same day.

Scores for catatonic motor disorder were obtained with subscores for 'positive' and 'negative' catatonic symptoms. Items not felt to be adequately classifiable as 'positive' or 'negative' were excluded. Where there was any doubt about whether individual items might rate extrapyramidal symptoms in some cases, 'narrow' positive and negative scores were derived by excluding these. Scores for tardive dyskinesia and parkinsonism were obtained on the same principle. Since some items on the tardive dyskinesia scale used could be confounded with catatonic symptoms or were arguably non-dyskinetic, a 'narrow' tardive dyskinesia score was produced by excluding all such items. Different scores were correlated using Spearman's method. In addition, factor analysis of 18 of the 93 items of the Modified Rogers Scale was performed.

In the main group of 75 patients, the total extrapyramidal score, calculated as the sum of the tardive dyskinesia and parkinsonism scores for each patient, were highly significantly correlated with the total catatonic score. When tardive dyskinesia and parkinsonism, and 'positive' and 'negative' catatonic scores were separated, an even more striking pattern of association and dissociation was observed. Tardive dyskinesia and 'positive' catatonic scores became even more significantly intercorrelated and there was a similar but less marked correlation between parkinsonism and 'negative' catatonic scores. The cross-correlations between tardive dyskinesia and 'negative', and parkinsonism and 'positive' catatonic scores were insignificant or inverse.

When the same analysis was repeated using the strictest narrow catatonic ratings and strictest narrow tardive dyskinesia scores and parkinsonism scores, the correlation between narrow positive catatonic and narrow tardive dyskinesia, and between narrow negative catatonic and parkinsonism, remained significant. When, to make sure that the intercorrelations were not merely an artefact of their mutual correlation with extraneous variables, the data were analysed using partial correlation techniques to control for the factors of age, chronicity and severity of illness, the correlations were hardly altered and there was no loss of significance. When, to try and eliminate any possible bias from simultaneous rating, the examinations were repeated under more rigorously blind conditions, the same pattern of correlations was found.

Factor analysis of 18 items covering both extrapyramidal and catatonic disorders, carried out on the 93 ratings on the Modified Rogers Scale produced two factors which together cumulatively accounted for nearly half the variance. The first factor, accounting for 32% of the variance, loaded principally on 'hyperkinetic' phenomena. The second, accounting for 17% of the variance, contained predominantly 'hypokinetic' phenomena. Both these factors tapped an admixture of extrapyramidal and catatonic abnormalities.

This study therefore found a highly significant clinical association between catatonic symptoms and extrapyramidal side-effects from neuroleptic medication in 93 patients at various stages of their schizophrenic illnesses, which survived a variety of attempts to make it disappear. Unless these patients' catatonic symptoms were mainly side-effects of neuroleptic medication or their extrapyramidal symptoms simply manifestations of the disease process of schizophrenia, the only reasonable explanation of the findings is interaction between drug and disease process.

The 'conflict of paradigms' hypothesis seems vindicated by this study with significant implications for the motor disorder of psychiatric illness. The contribution of neuroleptic medication to motor disorder in psychiatric patients cannot be considered in isolation from the motor disorder of the illnesses being treated. The only reason preventing such a view being generally accepted would seem to be preservation of the psychological paradigm for psychiatric disorder.

7 Posture, Tone and Motor Performance

POSTURE AND TONE

Friern study

In the Friern study of patients with severe psychiatric illness (Rogers 1985), 86 of the 100 patients currently had a disorder of posture. This was characteristically a tendency to flexion associated with various degrees of rigidity and typically affecting the head and neck.

- Altogether 72 patients, while supine, had a flexed posture of the head, tilting the face away from the horizontal towards their feet, persisting despite lack of support between bed and head; in 47 it was sustained during the whole period of observation. For 63 patients, while sitting, standing or walking, they had a flexed posture of the head, tilting the face away from the vertical towards the ground; in six the face was almost horizontal; in four it was associated with tilting of the head to one side; in 18 it was present during one period of examination but not another. In 37 patients, there was a marked dorsal kyphosis, typically of the upper dorsal spine. For 21 patients, while standing or walking, they had a flexed posture of one or both arms at the elbow, without the arms being crossed or the hands joined; in two there was a fixed flexion deformity of one or both elbows.
- In 21 patients there was a flexed posture of one or more of the fingers of one or both hands, typically of the little, ring and middle fingers with extension of the index (the pointing sign of Hunter), but in six with flexion at the metacarpo-phalangeal and extension at the interphalangeal joints; in nine there were fixed flexion deformities, typically of the little, little and ring, or little, ring and middle fingers.
- In 22 patients while standing or walking, they had an exaggerated lumbar lordosis (8); hyperpronation, abduction, or both of one or both arms (6); hyperextension, abduction or both of the fingers of one or both hands (11); or a combination of these. In 20 of the 22, this was associated with a flexed posture of the head.
- In 11 patients, there was a tendency for postures to persist after active or passive movements, varying from persistent extension of the legs at the knee after sitting down heavily in a low chair, to persistence in the upper limbs of

inappropriate postures set by the least pressure from one of the examiner's fingers, but in none persisting for more than a few seconds.

● A total of 71 patients had increased neck tone when supine, which was marked in 13, and 45 had increased tone of the arm at the elbow, which was marked in four. In 43 there was increased tone at both sites. Only two had decreased neck and arm tone. When sitting or standing, there was increased neck tone, compared to that when lying down, in 45 and decreased tone in only one.

● When upright, 78 patients had increased neck tone, which was marked in 31 and none had decreased tone; 45 had 'cogwheeling' (repeated, ratchet-like increase in tone) on passive movements of neck or arms; eight had 'gegenhalten' (increase in tone proportional to strength of passive movement).

Altogether 55 of the patients had received neuroleptic medication within the previous 12 months ('current'), 37 had received neuroleptic medication but not in the previous 12 months ('previous') and eight had no record of ever having received any ('never'). This information was collected after all the clinical examinations were complete. The percentages of patients in the whole group of 100 patients and in each of these treatment subgroups with particular disorders of posture or tone are shown in Table 7.1. There was no marked association of this disorder of posture and tone with exposure to neuroleptic medication, although it was more common in those currently receiving this medication.

Before the use of neuroleptic medication in any patient in the hospital in 1954, 50 patients had been noted to have an abnormality of posture. The abnormality

Table 7.1 Percentage of patients with disorders of posture and tone within various neuroleptic treatment groups

Motor disorder	Whole group ($n = 100$) (%)	Current ($n = 55$) (%)	Previous ($n = 37$) (%)	Never ($n = 8$) (%)
Head flexion				
supine	72	75	73	50
upright	63	73	51	50
Dorsal kyphosis	37	44	30	25
Arm flexion	21	24	19	13
Finger flexion	21	25	19	0
Extension/pronation/				
abduction	22	27	16	13
Persistence of				
postures	11	15	5	13
Increased neck tone	71	82	59	50
Increased arm tone	45	55	35	25
Cogwheeling	45	42	49	50
Gegenhalten	8	11	5	0

of posture was often not specified with descriptions, such as adopting attitudes or simply attitudinising, but in 28 patients, flexion postures were described such as 'lying with head off the pillow', 'holds herself rigid and lies doubled up with knees on chest', 'sits for long periods in a state of extreme flexion', 'remains through the interview with his chin resting on his sternum', 'stands totally immobile in a fixed stooping attitude and quite immovable facies', 'stands with "Neanderthal" posture', 'shuffles into the examination room with a somewhat parkinsonian attitude and gait', 'stands with her head bent on her chest and her left hand is partially closed; any effort to open it is resisted; the middle, ring and little fingers are kept flexed'; 16 patients had persistence of postures or waxy flexibility.

Of the 50 patients with abnormality noted before 1955, in 19 at least one of the observations was made on first admission to a long-stay psychiatric hospital, and in 29 within five years of first admission; 47 currently had one or more of the abnormalities of posture described. Abnormality of posture, therefore, was not always present at the beginning of the illness but, once present, tended to be permanent.

Of the total 100 patients: 34 were first admitted between 1907 and 1926; 33 between 1927 and 1935; and 33 between 1936 and 1955. Of the 50 patients with abnormality of posture noted before 1955: 17 were first admitted between 1907 and 1926; 15 between 1927 and 1935; and 18 between 1936 and 1955. Disorder of posture was thus distributed fairly evenly among patients with a case-note diagnosis of schizophrenia admitted to the hospital over a 50-year span.

Disorder of tone was noted before 1955 in 14 patients, who were noted to have rigidity or resistiveness.

Other studies

The disorder in the Friern patients matches the classic abnormalities of posture and tone in catatonic schizophrenia described by Marsden et al. (1975) in their review of psychiatric motor disorders. In this review, abnormal postures are included in the category of stereotypy and mannerism:

Stereotyped postures refer to awkward and sometimes bizarre body positions that are maintained for long periods of time. Examples included lying in bed with the head elevated as if on a 'psychological pillow', lying with the knees drawn up to the chin, or sitting with the upper and lower portions of the body twisted at right angles. Manneristic postures, by contrast, are said to be less rigidly maintained and usually are caricatured exaggerations of more normal positions (Marsden et al. 1975).

Abnormal tone is included under automatic obedience and negativism:

Automatic obedience is characterised by an abnormal degree of compliance and is manifested by a variety of abnormal postures, the best known of which is 'waxy flexi-bility' or catalepsy, a relatively uncommon disturbance in which an individual allows himself to be placed in awkward positions that are maintained for long periods. Variations of this unusual disturbance include mitgehen, in which a body part continues to move in a given direction in response to light pressure applied by the examiner, or cooperation, in which the displaced body part springs back to its original position when released . . . Muscle tone is quite variable and, although often increased, the clenched fist or fixed jaw and head position frequently described differs considerably from the more generalised rigidity of extrapyramidal disease. Muscle tone in the limbs or trunk is actually quite inconstant and may increase only in response to attempts to manipulate the patient. Occasionally tone may be extremely flaccid (Marsden et al. 1975).

A more detailed description of this disorder was given by Dide et al. (1921). They described flexion of the head, whether the patient was standing or sitting, with the chin touching the chest, eyes half shut and directed towards the ground, dorsal kyphosis typically at the level of the upper dorsal spine, adduction of the arms, which were flexed at right angles at the elbows, and flexion of the fingers except for extension of the thumb. There was no swing of the arms when they walked. A resting tremor was unusual. Increased tone was a constant feature, whether at rest or on movement or during persistence of passively produced postures. The increased tone was present in all muscle groups but was more marked in flexor muscles. Catalepsy, or the persistence of passively induced postures, was most marked the nearer the imposed posture was to spontaneous flexion postures. These features were not necessarily progressive or irreversible except for ankylosis secondary to abnormal postures, producing, for example, permanent dorsal kyphosis. They called this motor disorder the parkinsonian syndrome of schizophrenia to draw attention to the parallelism with post-encephalitic motor disorder.

Figure 4(a), showing flexion of the trunk leading to permanent kyphosis in a patient with schizophrenia, is taken from Bleuler's own account of schizophrenia in his 1923 *Textbook of Psychiatry* (Bleuler 1923). This flexion posture of the trunk was similar to post-encephalitic disorder as shown in Figure 4(b) (Martin 1983), which could also lead to permanent kyphosis as shown in Figure 4(c), an unpublished illustration from Steck's study of extrapyramidal disorders in psychiatric illness (Steck 1926, 1927).

Following the interest of investigators such as Dide and Steck, however, the implications of this parallelism were not followed up as neurology and psychiatry advanced with hardly any cross-fertilisation, despite obvious parallel in the motor disorders considered in each discipline. Figure 5(a) shows reversible flexion of the head in a patient with chronic schizophrenia, one of the 18 of the 100 patients in the Friern study who showed this feature. The patient shown spent most of the day looking at the ground. If asked, however, he could look up as shown. This is a recognised and classic feature of schizophrenia, which has usually been given a psychosocial explanation in terms of psychological withdrawal or institutional-isation. It is, however, similar to postural disorder found in post-encephalitic patients, as shown in Figure 5(b), an illustration from Purdon Martin's 1962 *Lancet* article on this disorder (Martin et al. 1962).

If neurology was slow to appreciate the relevance of basal ganglia pathology to postural disorder (Martin 1983), psychiatry has been even slower. Papers such as the Martin et al. 1962 Lancet paper, contain interesting and obvious parallel with the postural disorder of patients with severe psychiatric illness but I am unaware of any reference to this paper in the psychiatric literature.

Flexion deformities of the fingers provide another of these parallels. This was present in 21 of the 100 psychiatric patients in the Friern study. It was a classic feature of schizophrenia, as shown in Figure 6(a) taken from Jelliffe and White's (1917) textbook, where it is described as a mannerism. Parkinsonism, especially post-encephalitic, was also associated with flexion deformities of the extremities which could result in contractures: Figure 6(b) is taken from a recent paper by Kyriakides and Hewer (1988). Such postural abnormalities of the hands in post-encephalitic patients were reversible, at least in the initial stages, during sleep-walking (Nielson 1936), just as severe flexion postures and waxy flexibility in catatonic patients were shown to disappear during sleep (Forbes 1934).

Catalepsy, or waxy flexibility, the classic abnormality of tone in catatonia has not been the subject of detailed study since investigations such as those of Claude & Baruk (1928). Gegenhalten or 'counter-pull', however, another 'psychiatric' abnormality of tone shown by eight patients in the Friern study, has recently been described in various neurological disorders (Tyrrell & Rossor 1988). Gegenhalten was defined by Kleist as 'a pure motor negativism resisting changes of position, such that any attempt to change the position of a limb, or part of the body, by passive movement is met by a muscular tension which increases as the examiner changes his force, that is an active resistance to changes of position'. Kleist emphasised that it was not a general 'negativism'. It only affected certain limbs or muscle groups, particularly the adductors of upper and lower limbs, and could be elicited by repeated movements of muscles where it was not initially obvious. He described it in various disorders including catatonia and arteriosclerotic disease. The instruction to relax could exacerbate the rigidity. Tyrrell and Rossor describe this phenomenon in 10 patients with Alzheimer's disease, cerebro-vascular disease or cerebrodegenerative disease. In four patients, the rigidity became more pronounced after the instruction to relax. In nine patients, there was an association with dyspraxia on verbal command, and they suggested that gegenhalten could be viewed as ideomotor dyspraxia.

MOTOR PERFORMANCE

Friern study

In the Friern study (Rogers 1985), on current examination, 97 of the 100 patients had an abnormality of purposive movement. This was characterised by difficulty with the initiation, efficient execution of, or persistence with purposive motor activity. It resulted in restriction of the motor repertoire available to them in particular stimulus situations.

- Forty-seven were generally underactive, for example sitting all day doing nothing, going back to bed if allowed, or standing in 'poses' for long periods.
- Eighty-two needed help or encouragement with washing or dressing, and 26 of these with eating, for example, to use the right utensils, or needing the spoon to be placed in their hand to start them off.
- In 37 patients there was a marked reduction of spontaneous motor activity, apart from abnormal movements of the extremities.
- Ten had akinetic episodes—abrupt, temporary cessation of spontaneous movements, lasting up to several seconds, interrupting the flow of normal or abnormal movements, which could be accompanied by deviation of the head and eyes.
- There was slowness of spontaneous movements, as in a slow running film, in six patients; while five performed spontaneous movements abruptly.

On testing for elicited movement—pursuit eye movements, closing the eyes, protruding the tongue, elevating the arms, performing 'piano-playing' movements of the fingers (with demonstration), getting up and sitting down—the following was found:

- Only eight performed the eye, oro-facial and upper limb movements without difficulty.
- Thirteen had no difficulty with the pursuit eye movements.
- Nineteen had no difficulty with the upper limb movements.
- Thirty-four had no difficulty with the oro-facial movements.
- 43 patients did not attempt any of these movements at all, but 13 of these, when asked to stand, sit or walk, did so.

To test for echopraxia, before asking for any movements to be performed, the examiner extended one hand and then the other, as if to shake hands, and then raised either arm and forefinger in turn. When the examiner's right hand was extended to each patient, 82 extended theirs; when his left hand was extended, 62 extended theirs. In response to elevation of the arms or forefingers, 29 raised their arms and 15 their forefingers.

The percentages of patients in the whole group of 100 patients and in each of the neuroleptic treatment subgroups with particular disorders of purposive movement are shown in the Table 7.2. Again there was no marked association of these disorders with the use of neuroleptic medication. Before the introduction of neuroleptic medication in 1954, 83 of the 100 patients were noted to have an abnormality of purposive movement, in 25 before first psychiatric admission, with descriptions such as 'dull, retarded and anergic', 'perpetually languid, restricted in interests and devoid of initiative', 'her movements are slow', 'slow in response to questions and slow in motor activity', 'often motionless', 'stands with his head

Table 7.2 Percentage of patients with disorders of purposive movement within various neuroleptic treatment groups

Motor disorder	Whole group ($n = 100$) (%)	Current ($n = 55$) (%)	Previous ($n = 37$) (%)	Never ($n = 8$) (%)
Help washing/dressing	82	80	89	63
General underactivity	47	45	49	50
Impaired elicited face or arm movements	38	36	41	38
Reduced spontaneous movements	37	33	43	38
Echopraxia for arm elevation	29	25	27	63
Akinetic episodes	10	11	8	13

down, never moves, never speaks', 'sits immobile throughout day, except when moved, but can be got to dance', 'the spoon has to be placed in her hand to start her off with her meals and she has to be initiated at night before she makes any attempt to go to bed', 'gazes at one part of a newspaper for hours at a time', 'even when a pin is stuck in his arm, he makes no effort to extract it'.

Of these 83 patients, in 57 at least one of the observations was made on or before first admission and in 72 within 5 years of first admission; 81 currently had one or more of the abnormalities of purposive movement described. Disorder of purposive movement, therefore, was present in the majority of these 100 patients from quite an early stage of their illnesses and tended to be permanent.

Other studies

Like other motor disorders in psychiatric patients, impairment of motor performance has been open to various interpretations. Forty years ago, psychological interpretations were prevalent. When, for example, catatonic patients were observed to play ball, when they could otherwise hardly move, one explanation offered was:

> Ball-playing is communication but communication at a distance, and, as play without rules and aims, it is a communication and partnership without obligations and consequences (Straus & Griffith 1955).

On the other hand, in a series of studies before the introduction of neuroleptic medication, not primarily aimed at assessment of motor function but rather at the effects on psychological function of removal of frontal cortical tissue from the brain, King (1954) found that disturbances of psychomotor function could be demonstrated in chronic mental patients. He used tests of reaction time as a measure of the speed of initiating movement, speed of tapping as a measure of speed in stereotyped movement, and finger dexterity as a measure of speed in manual dexterity and precision. The degree of psychomotor disturbance was related to the clinical estimate of severity of illness. It was most marked in patients with chronic schizophrenia. He felt that the psychomotor retardation shown by these patients formed part of their schizophrenic disorder, and came to the conclusion that psychomotor disorder was a fundamental part of psychiatric disorders.

Other authors drew attention to the similarity of impairment of motor perform-ance, such as perseveration, the non-purposeful continuation of an act, sensation or idea, which occurred in neurological conditions such as delirium, brain injury, dementia, epilepsy as well as psychiatric disorders such as schizophrenia (Freeman & Gathercole 1966), but at this time a psychological paradigm was still common for both psychiatric and neurological motor disorder. Impersistence in patients with hemiplegia, for example, was regarded by some as a compulsive disorder, inability to keep the eyes closed being compulsive eye opening, and to keep the mouth open, compulsive mouth closure (Berlin 1955).

In their consideration of spontaneous movement disorders in psychotic patients, Marsden et al. (1975) clearly separated psychiatric and neurological motor dis-order. They described akinetic features of catatonic schizophrenia, including lack of spontaneity, expressionless facies, transient bursts of activity in akinetic patients, sudden blocking or transient akinetic episodes. In its most severe form, catatonic stupor, the patient sat or lay motionless with fixed, expressionless facies and resisted all efforts at communication or mobilisation. Although these features all had their counterparts in Parkinson's syndrome, they insisted that the simi-larities were limited to external appearances, the motor disorder in the schizo-phrenic patients being secondary to abnormal mental states, such as negativism, which had no counterpart in Parkinson's disease.

One of the most widely used scales for assessing impairment of motor perform-ance in psychiatric disorder is the SANS (Scale for the Assessment of Negative Symptoms) developed by Nancy Andreasen (1989a). This consists of ratings for unchanging facial expression, decreased spontaneous movements, paucity of expressive gestures, poor eye contact, affective non-responsivity, lack of vocal inflections, poverty of speech, poverty of content of speech, blocking, increased latency of response, grooming and hygiene, impersistence at work or school, physical anergia, recreational interests and activities, sexual interest and activity, ability to feel intimacy and closeness, relationships with friends and peers, social inattentiveness, inattentiveness during mental status testing and global ratings for affective flattening, avolition–apathy, anhedonia–asociality and attention. Although Andreasen believed that all the signs and symptoms of schizophrenia must ultimately reflect neural activity in the brain (Andreasen 1989b), she stopped short of a neurological framework for making sense of the symptoms on her scale.

The lack of a neurological approach led to apparently puzzling findings. Goode et al. (1981) reported setting out to investigate impairment of fine motor performance produced by anti-psychotic medication in patients with schizo-phrenia and schizo-affective disorder. They found, contrary to their expectations, significant deficits in fine motor performance in untreated patients compared to controls and improvement in performance after medication. This report was followed by further studies confirming that impairment of fine motor per-formance in schizophrenic patients was improved by neuroleptic medication (Vrtunski et al. 1989).

A neurological approach is now more and more common. Manschreck et al. (1982) examined 37 patients with schizophrenia and 16 with affective disorder for abnormality of voluntary motor activity. Only one schizophrenic patient was subtyped as catatonic. All patients were of average pre-morbid intelligence, aged between 18 and 60 years of age and free of any neurological or medical illness. Of the schizophrenic patients, 30 were receiving neuroleptic medication, as were 10 affective patients. Voluntary motor behaviour was evaluated by observation of spontaneous motor anomalies and performance of elicited skilled movements. Extrapyramidal motor disorder, including tardive dyskinesia, was assessed with two rating scales, including the AIMS. Neurological 'soft' signs, features of thought disorder and affective blunting were also assessed. Disturbance of volun-tary motor activity was found in 29 of the 30 schizophrenic patients but infrequently in the affective group. Scores of medicated and non-medicated schizophrenic patients for motor performance were significantly different, being better in medicated subjects. Disturbance of voluntary motor disorder was associated with affective blunting, soft neurological signs and, most strikingly, with thought disorder. The authors suggested that disturbance in voluntary motor activity, not attributable to drug effect or known neurological disorder, occurs in virtually all cases of conservatively defined schizophrenia, and that certain motor abnormalities and thought disorder in schizophrenic patients could have a common pathogenetic basis. The same group (Manschreck et al. 1985) showed that deficient motor synchrony in schizophrenic patients was associated with nega-tive features of the schizophrenic disorder and again that this performance was worse in unmedicated as opposed to medicated patients.

Others have suggested that lack of initiation of spontaneous movements, reduced motor activity and episodes of immobility may be fundamental defi-ciencies in other psychiatric disorders, such as depression with and without clinical retardation (Royant-Parola et al. 1986). A neurological approach leads to explora-tion of the neurophysiological basis for such impairment in different disorders. Guenther and his colleagues in Munich (Guenther et al. 1988), having described a 'psychotic motor syndrome' found in schizophrenic and depressed patients con-sisting of disturbances of lip and tongue movements, fine and gross movements of the dominant hand and impaired complex motor co-ordination of the extremities, have performed cerebral blood flow and electro-encephalograph (EEG) studies to explore the cerebral dysfunction underlying this motor disorder.

Echo phenomena, the automatic repetition of others' actions (echopraxia) or words (echolalia), represents disorder of motor performance extending into behaviour disorder. It can be a feature of certain cases of clouded consciousness of various origins, aphasia, dementia, mental handicap, epilepsy, and catatonic states including schizophrenia, as well as being found in normal childhood development and states of fatigue and lack of attention in normal subjects. Again it has been open to various interpretations. Psychodynamic explanations of echo phenomena, for example, in terms of their 'mocking function', have been offered (Carluccio et al. 1964). In schizophrenic illness it has been considered as an adaptation serving as a primitive form of sensori-motor communication in interpersonal situations (Chapman & McGhie 1964). Explanation of echo phenomena in schizophrenic patients in terms of bizarre delusions and hallucinatory experiences continues to be conventional (Ford 1989).

Still the best paper on echo phenomena is that of Stengel (1947). He showed that the phenomenon is not an indiscriminate automatic repetition, but depended on the specific setting and unlike other repetitive disorders of speech or action, such as the automatic repetition of the subject's own actions (palipraxia) and words (palilalia), had a fundamental social nature. He described, for example, aphasic patients where understanding of spoken language was almost completely lost so that they could not repeat spoken language to request but who showed marked echolalia. This only occurred, however, when they were addressed in conversation. If the examiner turned his back and spoke to himself or to someone else, however loudly or slowly, there was no echoing, but if the patient's eyes were covered so that they could not see whether or not they were being addressed, it did occur.

Stengel saw echo phenomena as a vindication of Hughling Jackson's contention that there is no antithesis between the automatic and voluntary as far as motor activity is concerned, but that there are only degrees from the 'most automatic' to the 'least automatic' or voluntary. Echo phenomena were examples of the transition from the automatic to the almost voluntary and purposeful. In the Friern study, echopraxia was triggered in a certain number of patients by socially non-meaningful stimuli, such as finger or arm raising, but in a greater proportion by the more meaningful stimulus of hand extension, the normal cue for shaking hands. The behavioural reflex called echopraxia, shown as a release phenomenon in these patients, could well be an important constituent of the normal handshake and other motor manifestations of social behaviour.

STUPOR AND AKINESIA

Psychiatric psychomotor retardation and neurological akinesia and akinetic mutism are an *experimentum crucis* of the 'conflict of paradigms' hypothesis, which predicts that they are indistinguishable.

According to Berrios (1981), the psychiatric concept of stupor, the symptom complex whose central feature is a reduction or absence of action and speech, has passed through distinct evolutionary stages. During the first stage, starting with the Greeks, stupor was regarded as a simple state of non-responsiveness. During the second stage, starting in the 1840s, the analysis of intrapsychical content was considered essential to diagnosis. Baillerger, a French psychiatrist, developed the first 'psychiatric' conception of stupor, with depressive stupor the archetype. The third stage, starting in the last decade of the nineteenth century, saw the completion of the 'psychologisation' of the stupors, with stupor interpreted as psychological inhibition or regression. This view for a long time overshadowed the fourth stage, starting at the turn of the century, viewing stupor as a primary disorder of motility, exemplified by Wernicke, who coined the term 'akinesia'.

Akinesia can be defined as difficulty with the initiation, efficient execution of, and persistence with purposive movement. Wernicke's new term 'akinesia' took over from a much older term 'abulia' to describe psychomotor retardation, slowness, apathy and lack of spontaneity, denoting lack or weakness of will, which was in common use before 1900. Auerbach, a German author, writing in 1921, commented that what had been called abulia in 1902 was called akinesia in 1920 (Fisher 1983). Wernicke's pupil, Kleist, continued to use the terms 'akinesia' and 'hypokinesia' for poverty of movement in psychiatric disorder, as in catatonic schizophrenia, but following the epidemic of encephalitis lethargica, starting in 1917–18, the term 'akinesia' was gradually adopted by neurologists, together with the term 'bradykinesia' coined by Cruchet (1921), describing a general slowness of movement, comparable to a slow motion film, which again was a characteristic feature of the motor impairment following epidemic encephalitis.

The motor impairment of akinesia was not a simple one. Movements and actions could be perfectly possible on some occasions and completely impossible at other times. Abrahamson and Rabiner (1924) described encephalitic patients who during the day were rigid, immobile and unable to feed themselves, but at night were entirely relaxed, could walk about with ease and sometimes dance. Others were normally so rigid that in attempting to walk they would topple and crash down like a statue falling form a pedestal, but at other times, when visitors came, for example, they could entertain them with Russian dances that called for great agility, rapidity of movement and suppleness. Yet others would at times have a typical parkinsonian tremor, gait and posture with mask-like face and slow, monotonous voice and at other times be suddenly free of rigidity and run along with normal voice and no tremor. This 'on–off' phenomenon is now not uncommon in levodopa-treated patients with parkinsonism.

Some neurologists, such as Kinnier Wilson, maintained a neuropsychiatric approach to akinesia. In his 1925 Croonian lectures on disorders of motility and muscle tone (Wilson 1925), he pointed out that a very large part of every 'voluntary' movement is both 'involuntary' and 'outside consciousness'. Akinesia could not be ascribed to dysfunction of the corpus striatum alone but could arise at different neurophysiological levels in Hughlings Jackson's sense. Psychotic catatonic stupor and some of the akinesia of parkinsonism could be related to disorder at the highest physiological level, producing absence or diminution of the will to act or lack of central impulses. It took only a 'flip of the psychiatric Necker cube', however, to consider this unwillingness to move psychological rather than nerophysiological and exclude a neurophysiological approach to psychiatric disorder.

Many neurologists after Wilson avoided any consideration of 'higher' neurophysiological processes at all. Difficulty with movement in parkinsonism, for example, was considered a simple corollary of muscular rigidity and this continued to be the view of some eminent neurologists as late as the 1950s. Sir Francis Walshe, for example, writing in a volume to commemorate the bicentenary of James Parkinson's birth (Walshe 1955), maintained that 'abolishing rigidity restores the normal range and speed of movement and there is no necessity to invoke unknown factors to account for characteristic slowness and limitations of range of movement'.

After the introduction in the 1960s of levodopa, which had a dramatic effect on the symptoms of parkinsonism and especially akinesia, akinesia became accepted as a definite neurological symptom in its own right. Schwab and Zieper 1965), describing akinesia as the most devastating symptom of Parkinson's disease, defined it as impairment in initiating, continuing and altering voluntary movements. It appeared as soon as the Parkinson's disease process becomes bilateral. There was no association with the amount of rigidity and tremor. It could be made much worse by minor emotional stresses and unexpected sensory stimuli but could become considerably reduced under the stimulation of increased motivation and incentive. Under extraordinary stimulation, there could be complete but short-lived loss of akinesia, called akinesia paradoxica. Akinesia is now accepted as one of the major motor symptoms of parkinsonism and even by some as the core symptom of parkinsonism, as in the recent United Kingdom Parkinson's Disease Society brain bank diagnostic criteria for Parkinson's disease (Rogers et al. 1987).

In 1941, Cairns et al. (1941) described a severe form of akinesia. They described a patient in whom a cyst distending the third ventricle produced mutism, loss of voluntary and emotional movement, with the exception of movement of the eyeballs, and apparent loss of emotional feeling, which they called akinetic mutism. The symptoms disappeared almost immediately, and repeatedly, on aspiration of the cyst. Cairns suggested that these symptoms were due to a disturbance of the diencephalon affecting cortical function. This neurological concept of akinetic mutism subsequently became firmly established. Magoun (1950), in his description of the brainstem reticular activating system compared Cairns' case and the encephalitic syndrome described by von Economo (1931), to the effects of brainstem injury in experimental animals. These included as initial somnolence, lack of motor initiative, slowness, decreased activity, mutism and reduced facial mimetic activity. He described the diminution or absence of motor responsiveness, in animals and patients, as a lack of 'will' to move, or paralysis of volition rather than movement.

This came very close to contemporary descriptions of psychiatric catatonia. Sylvan Arieti, in his chapter on the functional psychoses in the American

Handbook of Psychiatry in 1959 (Arieti 1959) described the symptomatology of catatonia as consisting 'not of motor disorders but of will disorders. The patient cannot move, not because he is paralysed, but because he cannot will to move' (p. 468). He also appreciated that the catatonic type of schizophrenia could be confused with Cairns' akinetic mutism. In his 1952 review of disturbances of consciousness with lesions of the brainstem and diencephalon, Cairns (1952) likewise mentions a case of traumatic haemorrhage that produced a state of mutism, partial akinesia, catatonia and a certain amount of negativism, 'superficially resembling catatonic schizophrenia'. However, the similarity between these two syndromes did not arouse more than passing interest at this time. Neurology and psychiatry were divided by a conceptual chasm.

Clinical studies, however, repeatedly and invariably concluded that neurological akinetic mutism and psychiatric stupor were indistinguishable. Williams and Parsons-Smith (1951), in their investigation of thalamic activity in stupor, concluded that the clinical states called stupor by psychiatrists and akinetic mutism by neurologists were one and the same. They responded in the same way to intravenous barbiturates. Smith (1959) agreed that the term 'akinetic mutism' was used by neurologists to describe the stupor of psychiatrists. He described 27 cases, presenting as psychiatric first admissions, with immobility and muteness without loss of consciousness or organic paralysis. On investigation, no neurological or biochemical anomalies could be shown. The final diagnoses were depressive reaction in 12 cases, schizophrenia in nine, mixed neurotic states in four and epilepsy in two. Joyston-Bechal (1966) reviewed 100 of the 250 cases of stupor, defined as akinesis, mutism and relative preservation of consciousness, admitted to the Bethlem and Maudsley Hospitals between 1948 and 1961: in 18 of the patients it was total and in 82, partial. The absence of speech and movement was often temporarily in abeyance, either as a result of external stimulation or for no apparent reason; 31 had total amnesia for the period of stupor. The diagnoses, only possible after recovery from the stupor, were schizophrenia in 31, depression in 25, mixed neurotic in 10, organic in 20 and uncertain in 14. The features of the stupor were identical whether organically determined or not. Again he felt that akinetic mutism was equivalent to stupor.

One of the best 'pre-neurotransmitter era' reviews of akinetic mutism was provided by Klee (1961). The syndrome had been described in association with basilar artery thrombosis, narcolepsy, hydrocephalus, Wernicke's encephalopathy, encephalitis lethargica; tumours, infarction, haemorrhage and arteriovenous malformations of the midbrain and thalamus; bilateral destruction of the cingulate gyri due to infarction or tumour, and frontal lobe trauma, as well as in patients with various psychiatric disorders including schizophrenia, mania, depression and hysteria. Despite the various terms for the phenomenon used in different reports, the case histories he reported seemed to Klee to indicate that all the disturbances of speech and movement described were variations of the same basic disorder: an inhibition of motor function, comprising speech, movement and facial expression, with preservation of sensory functions and awareness.

Variations in the degree of inhibition could occur from one minute to the next, and the inhibition could last from minutes to months. There was variable amnesia for the period of inhibition. Wilder Penfield in his recent Sherrington lecture (Penfield 1958) had suggested that the centrencephalic system of the higher brainstem he had described with Jasper in 1954 provided the physical basis for Hughlings Jackson's highest level of functional representation. Klee suggested that akinetic mutism represented an isolated paralysis of this centrencephalic system.

In his chapter on the clinical symptomatology of basal ganglia disease in the *Handbook of Clinical Neurology*, Denny-Brown (1968) described voluntary movement as the sum total of the various physiological effects that can initiate and direct movement. He defined what he called 'hypokinesia', rather than akinesia, as difficulty in the initiation of all willed movement, the result of defect in the integration of one or more of the many factors contributing to normal motor performance. Motor apraxia differed from hypokinesia only in that the difficulty in initiation of movement is related to a particular stimulus situation. Hypokinesia was the primary symptom of damage to the basal ganglia, but could be produced by damage of what he called the 'basal ganglionic system' extending from cortex down to sub-cortical structures; at its most severe it produced the state called 'akinetic mutism'. Apraxia was produced by impairment of a particular part of the more specialised cortical apparatus subserving the various factors that initiate movement.

Hicks and Birren (1970), reviewing research on psychomotor slowing in ageing, psychosis and brain damage, suggested that the same brain mechanisms underlay the slowing in all three groups, involving a cortical–sub-cortical system that was diffuse in location but specific as to structures. At the same time, Ajuriaguerra (1975), reviewing the literature on the possible cerebral localisation of akinesia, found that it suggested a similar cerebral system, since it could be produced by lesions close to the medial neuraxis anywhere from the frontal poles to the pons, including the cingulate gyri, septum, medial temporal lobes, thalamus, hypothalamus and midbrain. Akinesia is to be distinguished from the locked-in syndrome or bilateral brain pyramidal syndrome, with mute quadriplegia and preservation of consciousness and communication by ocular movements and blinks, produced by pathological changes bilaterally in ventral pontine, ventral midbrain, internal capsules or middle portions of the cerebral peduncles, sparing the reticular formation (Chia 1991).

Markham (1973) has suggested that certain aspects of akinesia could be due to a disturbance in the gain or amplification of sensory input. This would explain the sudden 'freezing' produced by an auditory, visual or tactile input, or release from immobility by, for example, a tap on the shoulder, found in some patients. Other specific stimuli used to overcome the difficulty in initiation of desired movement, included tapping themselves slowly on top of the head with the fingertips while slowly rotating the entire body, or taped march music carried around for the purpose (Aring 1962; McCarthy 1979). I have a parkinsonian patient who becomes 'glued' to the floor but then, on removing one shoe, strides off normally. Visual, auditory or tactile inattention with lateralised akinesia of the hemiface or limbs of one side of the body is described as neglect, with the most severe form of neglect producing bilateral akinesia and mutism (Watson et al. 1978; Damasio et al. 1980; Laplane & Degos 1983). All this strongly suggests a disturbance in the reticular system being able to produce akinesia.

Psychic akinesia has been described as a form of akinesia with no or only mild motor disorder (Laplane et al. 1984, 1989). The main features are inertia and loss of drive. The spontaneous psychic akinesia is reversible when the subject is stimulated. Cognitive capacity can be normal. Attention has been drawn to the similarities between this concept of psychic akinesia and the concept of bradyphrenia, described by Naville in the wake of epidemic encephalitis (Rogers 1986). Others have suggested that psychic akinesia represents a variety of bilateral intentional neglect, or a less severe expression of akinetic mutism (Starkstein et al. 1989). Laplane and his colleagues described it in patients with lesions in the lentiform nuclei of the basal ganglia, especially the pallidum, with possibly secondary hypometabolism of the pre-frontal cortex on position emission tomography (PET) scanning, as a result of anoxic or toxic encephalopathy. They suggest that some psychiatric disorders, such as schizophrenia and depression, can include a more or less reversible psychic akinesia and that, here too, this could be related to structural and physiological disturbances in the systems linking the frontal associative cortex and the basal ganglia.

Miller Fisher (1983) suggested that minor degrees of psychomotor retardation are widespread throughout different clinical disorders, and the fully developed syndrome, akinetic mutism, is only the tip of an important clinical iceberg. He describes the following as features of akinetic mutism of different severity:

- Lack of spontaneity of action; lack of spontaneity of speech for comment or question; lack of initiative; slowness and poverty of movement; mental slowness; apathy; inertia; indifference; disinterestedness; reduced vigour and energy; lack of enthusiasm; impaired concentration and attention; ease of distraction; 'thinking of something else'; and 'daydreaming'. After a question or command, the verbal or motor response is given after a delay varying from a second or so up to several minutes. Replies consist of one or two words and speech is monotonous, matter of fact, without expression and unembellished by extra comment. The voice is faint or soft and at times only a whisper. The patient may respond to only one question in four or five or ten, or may obey only one command of several; or instead of answering, there is only a very slight nod or shake of the head. Conversation may be possible by telephone which is not possible face to face. Perseveration may be prominent, and the same answers can be given to several successive questions.
- The patients have a reduced flow of thoughts. They are uncomplaining and express little in the way of needs or satisfaction. Yet, politeness may be retained. The face is impassive. Emotional expression and feeling are greatly

reduced. Animation is lacking. Reaction to loved ones is slight, and tearfulness is in abeyance. Smiling and laughter are lacking or limited. Patients
disclaim nervousness, worry, or tenseness. They lack insight into their illness
or state.

- Motor responses are slow and hesitant and the excursion of the movement is
small and perhaps partial. If the act is to be repetitive, it is halted prema-
turely. The ability to make an effort is reduced; patients procrastinate and fail
to pursue and complete their tasks. Acts such as squeezing the examiner's
hand may consist of brief, repetitive, tentative contractions rather than a
single firm act. The patient may chew and swallow slowly, and food remnants
may be present in the mouth hours after a meal. The limbs may be held in
one position unnecessarily long, for periods up to several minutes, or the
patient does not automatically correct an awkward or abnormal position.
There may be periods when the patient does not respond at all or the output
fluctuates. Patients may look at the examiner and not reply, giving the
impression of hostility, yet, when questioned, disclaim being angry. They
may turn over and face away from the examiner, an action usually interpreted
as uncooperative. Incontinence of bowel and bladder is common.

These excellent clinical descriptions are entirely congruous with the classic
descriptions of impairment of motor performance in different psychiatric disorders
reviewed in this book. Fisher suggested that the cerebral function whose deficiency
results in the syndrome of akinetic mutism could be regarded as a basic functional
brain system. This system did not currently have a universally accepted name but
might, in fact, subserve all impulse to action and its malfunction could be a
fundamental cause of slowing of function in the central nervous system. Psycho-
logically it might be described as 'motivation'. In terms of localisation, he
suggested a mesencephalo-frontal activating system, overlapping with but not
identical with the reticular activating system.

Since, by current definition, akinesia is a neurological disorder it only occurs in
neurological disorder such as parkinsonism. It is time that akinesia was accepted
once again as a neuropsychiatric phenomenons which occurs in both psychiatric
and neurological disorder, as was the case when Wernicke introduced the term.

8 Activity, Abnormal Movements and Speech Production

ACTIVITY

Friern study

In the Friern study of 100 patients with severe psychiatric disorder, 64 of the patients showed abnormal activity.

- Twenty-five had generally increased activity, pacing up and down or round and round or wandering aimlessly. This could occur in distinct episodes lasting hours to days, recurring from every few days to every few months, and could alternate with periods of general underactivity. During examination, 13 either paced or wandered up and down, or were unable to sit for any length of time without getting up.
- Thirty-six patients had 'outbursts' of activity lasting from seconds to minutes, recurring from continuously through the day, to once a day or less, their frequency being characteristic for each patient. Their form for each patient was also characteristic, typically involving shouting and swearing, combined in some patients with threatening behaviour and in a few with actual assaults on others. These outbursts could be situationally provoked or apparently spontaneous. They could appear on a background of general underactivity or overactivity.
- Persistent and characteristic abnormal behaviour, including touching or following people, touching or collecting things, self-mutilation, destroying things, stripping, or excessive washing and cleaning, was observed in 20 patients.

Only 55 of the patients had received neuroleptic medication within the previous 12 months ('current'), while 37 had received neuroleptic medication but not in the previous 12 months ('previous') and eight had no record of ever having received any ('never'). The percentages of patients in the whole group of 100 patients and in each of these treatment subgroups with particular disorders of activity are shown in Table 8.1. All disorders of activity were more common in those currently being treated with neuroleptic medication but were still present in the other treatment subgroups.

Before the introduction of neuroleptic medication in 1954, 84 patients had abnormal activity noted, in 26 before their first psychiatric admission; 48 were

Table 8.1 Percentage of patients with disorders of activity within various neuroleptic
             treatment groups

Motor disorder	Whole group (n = 100) (%)	Current (n = 55) (%)	Previous (n = 37) (%)	Never (n = 8) (%)
General overactivity	25	35	14	13
Outbursts of activity	36	45	27	13
Continual activity on examination	13	18	8	0

described as overactive with descriptions such as 'couldn't sit nowhere', 'can't sleep, can't rest, runs about like mad', 'in a state of continuous hyperactivity'; 51 were described as impulsive with outbursts such as 'sits unoccupied occasionally leaping in the air while hitting his head', 'on occasions impulsively jumps out of bed and rushes out into the corridor and can give no reason for this conduct'; 43 showed abnormal behaviour such as obsessional touching of objects, hoarding rubbish, eating clothing, rubbish or faeces, or covering their face and avoiding all contact with those around them.

Of the 84 patients with abnormal activity noted before 1955, in 52 at least one of the observations was made on or before first admission, and in 73 within 5 years of first admission. Only 52 currently had one or more of the abnormalities of activity described. Abnormal activity, therefore, was a feature in a majority of the 100 patients fairly early on in their illness, but was not necessarily a permanent feature.

Other studies

Studies of abnormal activity in psychiatric disorder have concentrated on affective disorder. Measurement of motor activity with monitoring devices has confirmed increased motor activity in manic states and decreased activity in depressed states in patients compared with their activity level when euthymic (Weiss et al. 1974; Wolff et al. 1985).

Attempts to compare increased activity in psychiatric illnesses with that in neurological disorders have been few. Kahn and Cohen (1934) described a syndrome they called 'organic drivenness', which they felt was due to brainstem pathology and had significance for clinical psychiatry. It consisted of marked general hyperkinesis with either choreiform or tic-like, myoclonic movements in face, trunk and extremities, marked inability or impossibility of remaining still even for a few seconds, abruptness and clumsiness of performance of even simple movements, and the explosive release of all voluntarily inhibited activity. This could be associated with distractibility and hypomanic mood disorder. It could be found in various encephalopathies, notably encephalitis lethargica where some affected individuals could literally 'roll themselves to death', and cerebral degenerative diseases. They did not present any post-mortem findings but described all the patients showing neurological signs indicating brainstem involvement. They accepted that similar disorder could be found with frontal lobe pathology. They felt there was an overlap with motor disturbances found in schizophrenia.

Abnormal behaviour is almost a hallmark of psychiatric disorder. There have been relatively few studies of behaviour disorder in psychiatric illness viewed as abnormal activity, and little attempt to relate these to abnormal activity with a known neurological basis.

In 1937–39, Kluver and Bucy described the behavioural syndrome following bilateral temporal lobectomy in rhesus monkeys, now named after them. This consisted of 'psychic blindness', strong tendencies to examine all objects orally, an irresistible impulse to touch, loss of normal anger and fear responses, and increased sexual activity. Sylvano Arieti, later to become editor of the *American Handbook of Psychiatry*, immediately realised the relevance of the behavioural syndrome described in animals by Kluver and Bucy to some of the behavioural disorders found in chronic schizophrenia. He published (Arieti 1945) a study of the 'quasineurologic' phenomena in 250 patients, all female with chronic schizophrenia, who had been hospitalised for 7–47 years. He described various abnormal behaviours including grabbing food at the sight of it, extreme rapidity of eating, grabbing every small object and putting it into the mouth, including crumbs, cockroaches, stones, rags, paper, wood, clothes, pencils and leaves. Attempts to swallow such objects as ink wells and teaspoons had been, he felt, mistakenly considered as suicidal attempts. Patients could seem insensitive to pain, temperature and taste sensation. Arieti pointed out the similarity of the patients' behaviour with the syndrome recently described by Kluver and Bucy, and that this suggested that the schizophrenic process was organic in nature.

This was followed by descriptions of the Kluver–Bucy syndrome in humans, consisting of visual agnosia, apathy and flattened affect, altered sexual orientation, hyper-metamorphosis (forced responding to environmental stimuli), hyper-orality and bulimia, associated with various cerebral disorders including herpes encephalitis, surgical amygdalotomy, post-traumatic encephalopathy, paraneoplastic limbic dementia, adrenoleucodystrophy, bilateral temporal infarction, Pick's and Alzheimer's disease, hypoglycaemia and toxoplasmic encephalitis (Lilly et al. 1983). Psychiatric authors then became reluctant to accept the Kluver–Bucy syndrome as a part of psychiatric illness. For example, a patient was recently reported (Clarke & Browne 1990) with a 36-year admission to a psychiatric hospital and a diagnosis of schizophrenia, who showed the Kluver–Bucy syndrome. Neurological investigation, including brain biopsy, was not able to provide a specific diagnosis. The authors felt that in view of the Kluver–Bucy syndrome, the patient's diagnosis should be one of organic psychotic disorder of unknown aetiology, rather than schizophrenia. The alternative, regarding schizophrenia as an organic psychotic disorder of unknown aetiology, as Arieti had suggested when he first reported the association, requires a switch of the psychiatric Necker cube.

Some authors are now attempting neurological interpretation of apparently bizarre behaviour in psychiatric patients. Outbursts of typically aggressive behaviour, for example, have been described as an episodic dyscontrol syndrome or 'limbic epilepsy' and are the subject of an increasing number of studies (Girgis & Kiloh 1980). Luchins (1990) has recently suggested that 'bizarre behaviour' in chronic schizophrenia including polydipsia, pacing, constant smoking, strange grooming patterns, hoarding, stereotypies and mannerisms could be ascribed to hippocampal abnormality, especially in the left hemisphere. Comparable behaviours in experimental animals are augmented by hippocampal lesions, stress, increased drive state or dopaminergic agents, and reduced by 6-hydroxydopamine lesions to the nucleus accumbens or anti-psychotic agents. He suggests that such repetitive behaviour may reflect the failure of hippocampus to modulate the impact of mesolimbic dopaminergic activity on the nucleus accumbens and thus on motor behaviour.

One of the most forward looking of twentieth-century neurologists in terms of understanding motor function subserving behaviour was Derek Denny-Brown (1950, 1958). He felt that the 'functions' currently attributed to the motor regions of the frontal cortex, pyramidal tract and various extrapyramidal motor structures in contemporary neurology and neurophysiology textbooks bore critical analysis little better than the 'faculties' plotted by the phrenologists early last century. He suggested that willed movement is in fact the learned ability of the organism to adapt movements that are primarily reflex. He contrasted two sets of behavioural reaction to the environment—instinctive grasping or exploration and instinctive avoiding. On the basis of experimental animal work he suggested that exploratory behaviour was subserved by parietal cortex and avoiding behaviour by frontal premotor, cingulate and temporal hippocampal cortex. Normal behaviour required a balance between these two opposing tendencies. Damage to the mechanism of either could release abnormal activity of the other. Exploratory behaviour could thus be released by frontal and temporal lesions, and avoiding behaviour by parietal lesions. Instinctive exploration he called frontal or magnetic apraxia and instinctive avoiding parietal or repellent apraxia.

Application of Denny-Brown's concepts has started to be applied to neurological disorders. Lhermitte (1983) has described the forced grasping and use of different utilitarian objects, such as cups and combs, when presented visually or tactilely to patients with unilateral or bilateral frontal lesions of various aetiology. He sees this phenomenon as an extension of the bilateral manual grasping behaviour or magnetic apraxia, due to the disinhibited action of parietal lobe function with frontal lesions, described by Denny-Brown. Mori and Yamadori (1989) have described loss of exploratory activities and rejection of environmental contact, characterised by exaggerated withdrawal movements and refusal to be touched on the lips and tongue resulting in difficulty in feeding, in patients with bilateral parieto-temporal strokes, comparing this to Denny-Brown's repellent or parietal apraxia.

Application of Denny-Brown's ideas to psychiatric behaviour disorder has hardly started.

ABNORMAL MOVEMENTS

Friern study

In the Friern study, I used a simple descriptive distinction between different abnormal movements, rather than conventional neurological and psychiatric terminology, to avoid a priori classification of these movements as neurological or psychiatric. Altogether, 67 of the patients showed one or more abnormal movements of the head, trunk, limbs or face:

- Twenty-nine had superfluous, brief, random movements of the head, upper limbs or trunk, which were often jerky in quality.
- Twenty-nine had superfluous, semi-purposeful movements of the head or upper limbs, typically 'searching' of the head and 'grooming' of the upper limbs.
- Twenty-six had superfluous rhythmic movements including nodding or shaking of the head, rocking of the pelvis, pacing on the spot, wringing of the hands and rubbing or pinching movements of the thumb and other fingers.
- Sixteen had tremors, postural of the arms or head in 12, and resting of the arms in four.
- Eight had complex tics, either deviation of the head and pantomime of the upper limbs associated with shouting, swearing, unintelligible or soundless speech, or repeated touching with one or both hands of the other limbs or face in a regular but not invariable sequence.
- Three had superfluous, relatively sustained, spasmodic movements of the head, trunk or limbs.
- Two gyrated when standing or walking.

An individual patient could have a combination of the movements described, either simultaneously: continual writhing of the head and trunk with continual grooming movements of the upper limbs, or on different occasions: a continual, marked resting tremor of the upper limbs on one occasion and continual, brief, random movements of these limbs on another.

- Fifty-two patients had spontaneous, discrete contractions of one or more facial muscles varying from rapid and transient to slow and sustained. One or both sides of the face could be affected: in 30 the frontalis muscle was involved; in 16, the orbicularis oculi; in nine the corrugator supercilii; in 16, the elevators of the angles of the mouth or upper lip; in six, the orbicularis oris; in 21, the platysma.

- Thirty-five had more fluid, superfluous, random movements of the peri-oral muscles, not associated with speech production: in 12 there were associated similar movements of the peri-ocular muscles; in 17 there were associated random movements of the jaw and tongue.
- Eleven had a marked lack of facial expression, which could be associated with the abnormal movements just described.
- Nine had other movements of the lips, jaw or tongue, including tremor, deviations of the jaw and darting protrusions of the tongue.

There was a tendency for these abnormal movements to be commoner in the 55 patients who had received neuroleptic medication within the previous 12 months ('current'), but they were almost as common in the 37 who had received neuroleptic medication but not in the previous 12 months ('previous') and in the eight who had no record of ever having received any ('never'): see Table 8.2.

Before the introduction of neuroleptic medication in 1954, 71 of the 100 patients were noted to show different abnormal movements of the head, trunk or limbs. Most were described as mannerisms, with only occasional greater detail such as 'very manneristic patient who all day grimaces and flings his arms about working his fingers like a choreic', 'exhibits insane athetoid movements', 'exhibits insane mannerisms, e.g. he grimaces, contorts his body', 'grossly manneristic, frequent tic-like movements of mouth, cheeks and head', 'she exhibits a strange, writhing, snake-like movement of the limbs combined with grimaces which strongly resemble a choreo-athetosis'.

Table 8.2 Percentage of patients with abnormal movements within various neuroleptic treatment groups

Abnormal movements	Whole group ($n = 100$) (%)	Current ($n = 55$) (%)	Previous ($n = 37$) (%)	Never ($n = 8$) (%)
Head, trunk and limbs				
brief, random	29	27	35	13
semi-purposeful	29	29	30	25
rhythmic	26	33	19	13
tremor	16	20	11	13
complex tics	8	2	16	13
sustained, spasmodic	3	4	3	0
Oro-facial				
spasmodic				
contractions	52	58	46	38
fluid, random	35	40	27	38
rhythmic, tremor,				
tics	9	7	14	0

Of these 71 patients: 21 were first admitted between 1907 and 1926; 25 between 1927 and 1935; and 25 between 1936 and 1955. In 18 of the 71, at least one of the observations was made on or before first admission, and in 49 within 5 years of first admission; 50 currently had one or more of the abnormal movements of head, trunk or limbs described.

Abnormal facial movements or postures had been noted in 77: 48 had grimacing; 36 inappropriate or 'schizophrenic' smiling; 22 fixed facial expressions; and 15 various movements, such as spasms, twitching, tic-like movements, screwing up of the eyes and pursing of the lips; 22 were described as having an expressionless face, 15 of these having abnormal movements or expressions noted at other times.

Of these 77 patients: 29 were first admitted between 1907 and 1926; 22 between 1927 and 1935; and 26 between 1936 and 1955. In 30, at least one of the observations was made on or before first admission, and in 56 within 5 years of first admission; 59 currently had one or more of the abnormal facial or oro-facial movements or postures described.

Abnormal movements of the head, trunk, limbs and face, therefore, were present from fairly early on in the majority of these 100 patients but were not necessarily a permanent feature.

Other studies

Interest in abnormal movements in psychiatric patients only really began after the introduction of neuroleptic medication in the 1950s. Before then abnormal movements in such patients were categorised mainly as stereotypies or mannerisms.

The term 'stereotypy' was introduced into psychiatry by Falret in 1864, some 10 years before Kahlbaum's formulation of catatonia (Guiraud 1936). Like 'mannerism', the other term used to describe psychiatric motor disorder, it was borrowed from the ordinary language of the time and exact definition of these terms was difficult. A modern definition is provided by Marsden and colleagues:

> . . . stereotypy refers to isolated, purposeless movements carried out in a uniform and repetitive way. Mannerism is distinguished from stereotypy as an unusual or bizarre way of carrying out purposeful activity that results from the incorporation of stereotypy into goal-directed acts. From a practical point of view, these two disorders usually occur together, making the distinction between them arbitrary. Stereotypy and mannerism may take the form of repetitive movements (hyperkinesia) or of persistent abnormal postures (hypokinesia). (Marsden et al. 1975):

A large number of different motor disorders can thus be included under these terms. A modern study of stereotypy in 13 chronic schizophrenic patients (Jones 1965), for example, includes as stereotypies a facial expression suggesting an affect of fear or embarrassment, sitting curled up in a foetal position and standing in a rigid posture. In keeping with the currently favoured psychological paradigm, Jones tried to examine the understandability of the stereotypies, but concluded that delusional ideas could be advanced as an adequate explanation of the patients' stereotyped behaviour in only one of the 12 cases. He showed that stereotypies were improved by an increased level of attention and worsened by anxiety. There was a marked variability in their form on longitudinal observations of individual patients over a 6-month period.

In mentally handicapped subjects, stereotyped movements can similarly vary markedly in different environmental situations and also in the same environmental situation at different times in the same subject (Baumeister et al. 1980). With severe mental handicap, motor activity can be almost restricted to stereotypies, hardly affected by environmental influences and seeming to have an inherent periodicity (Meier-Koll & Pohl 1979).

Brickner et al. (1940), in a very forward-looking paper in 1940, suggested that fixed repetitive behaviour could be placed on a continuum from perseveration through echolalia, palilalia and stereotypy of movement or thought to obsessive-compulsive disorder. They stressed the importance of distinguishing psychology and physiology, each with its own vocabulary but which often tended to become confused. The whole spectrum of different repetitive motor behaviours could be found in definite cerebral disorders. A uniform thread ran through the entire spectrum, suggesting a common underlying physiological mechanism for all of them. Ridley and Baker (1982) have recently revived the idea of repetitive movements lying on a spectrum from involuntary, 'neurological' movements such as tremor and chorea, through 'functionally autonomous' rhythmic or complex sequences of obscure purpose, or stereotypies, to rituals and obsessive-compulsive behaviour, and finally voluntary, skilled, learned movements. Stereotyped movements were found with constraint, such as in prison cells, social and sensory deprivation in infancy, amphetamine abuse and psychotic states. They suggested they were a consequence of failure to use sensory input to direct behaviour.

Frith and Done (1986) define stereotyped behaviour as any purposeless movement or act that occurs repeatedly. They point out that this definition includes, in neurological and psychiatric terminology, tremor, tics, dyskinesia, perseveration, stereotypy, mannerisms and obsessional phenomena. They thus abandon traditional distinctions between neurological and psychiatric motor disorder. Instead, they suggest that different abnormal movements can be analysed as to how they lie along different continua of severity which are not mutually exclusive:

- Complexity, the number of components involved in the movement or act, which can vary from a simple finger movement to flailing of the limbs.
- Co-ordination, the relationships between agonist and antagonist muscles, varying from random flailing of the limbs to a smooth 'goal directed' movement.
- Degree of conscious control, the distinction between voluntary and involuntary movements.

Large-scale studies of abnormal movements in psychiatric patients, although all carried out after the introduction of neuroleptic medication, suggest that a simple division into neurological movement disorders, presumed due to medication, and the psychiatric categories of stereotypy and mannerism is not possible. Jones and Hunter (1969) described the abnormal movements of 127 patients with chronic psychiatric illness. The patients had been selected by length of current admission to one district psychiatric hospital. Their average age was 64 years and the average length of hospitalisation was 36 years: 81% had a diagnosis of schizophrenia. A proportion of these patients later formed part of my 1978 Friern study of motor disorder (Rogers 1985). Altogether 66% of the 127 patients showed abnormal movements. These were classified into four groups: tremor, choreo-athetosis, including oral dyskinesia, tics and stereotypies, including trunk rocking, hand movements and oral movements. The study was presented at a workshop on psychotropic drugs. The prevalence of these movements was higher in those who had been treated with neuroleptic medication but the movements were present in patients who had never received such medication. They were found in 88% of 17 patients currently receiving neuroleptic medication, in 74% of 65 patients who had previously received it and in 49% of 45 patients who had no record of ever having received any. The abnormal movements had been observed in the patients in the earlier years of their illness before any neuroleptic medication had become available. The authors suggested that the disease process of 'functional psychosis' included neurological involvement. At the time, this was a novel suggestion. A discussant at the meeting offered a more conventional view. He argued that since the tics and repetitive movements described were regularly seen only in mental institutions, they had to be psychogenic in origin.

Shortly after this, Yarden and Discipio (1971) surveyed all consecutive first admissions over a 12-month period to a psychiatric unit that accepted all psychiatric referrals from its catchment area: 18 patients with a diagnosis of schizophrenia and abnormal movements were selected for prospective study. They were all currently drug-free, although some had had neuroleptic medication for short periods a few months before admission in mild or moderate doses. All were under age 37 years and none had a history of brain damage, mental handicap, clinical neurological illness or more than a total of 2 years previous hospitalisation. The abnormal movements observed were choreiform movements, athetoid movements, tics, stereotypies and mannerisms. A control group of patients, matched for all these features except the presence of abnormal movements was selected by examining the next two consecutive admissions to each trial subject, making 36 control patients in all.

Psychiatric and neurological examinations of these subjects were carried out at 6-monthly intervals for some 3 years. The schizophrenic patients with abnormal movements, compared to those without, had a significantly earlier onset of illness, were younger at first hospitalisation and went on to develop a steadily progressive deterioration with nearly twice as much total hospitalisation altogether. They had more severe clinical features, notably of impairment of speech production, purposeless activity, negativism and neglect of personal hygiene. They were little affected by medication or other treatment, and if they could be discharged from hospital needed full-time care.

The authors felt that these schizophrenic patients with choreiform and other hyperkinetic abnormal movements created an impression of organic impairment since their movement disorders were reminiscent of heredo-degenerative disorders of the basal ganglia and their thinking and speech was so grossly affected that they appeared demented. They suggested that there was probably an overlap in pathogenesis between such patients and Huntington's chorea, chronic manganese poisoning, the levodopa induced psychosis/dyskinesia complex, and phenothiazine-induced tardive dyskinesia.

In Owens et al.'s study (1982), a group of 510 patients hospitalised with chronic schizophrenia, according to the Feighner criteria and Present State Examination, which excludes diagnosable neurologic disorders, showed a prevalence of abnormal movements of 50.4%. Subsequent scrutiny of the case notes disclosed that 65 of these patients had no record of ever having received neuroleptic medication, probably representing the largest group of schizophrenic patients untreated with neuroleptic medication examined for motor disorder in recent times. When the patients with no history of neuroleptic treatment were compared to those with a history of treatment, there was a close similarity in the prevalence, severity, and distribution of abnormal involuntary movements in both groups, although the prevalence of abnormal movements was higher in the treated patients. They concluded that spontaneous involuntary disorders of movement could be a feature of severe, chronic schizophrenia unmodified by neuroleptic drugs, and that a pathological cerebral process underlay at least some cases of severe, chronic schizophrenia.

ABNORMAL EYE MOVEMENTS AND BLINKING

Friern study

Of the 100 patients in the Friern study, 48 had abnormal spontaneous eye movements, and 38 an obvious abnormality of blinking

- Twenty-eight had sudden, spontaneous conjugate deviation of the eyes, which could be brief and darting or sustained for up to several seconds. The head was often deviated in the same direction. This was most commonly up and lateral, but could be up, lateral or down and lateral. The deviation could be associated with outbursts of speech or arrest of speech and movement.
- Twenty-six had random, roving conjugate eye movements, typically associated with 'searching' semi-purposeful movements of the head. When associated with head flexion and wandering it produced an impression of 'looking for a lost sixpence'.
- Three had fixity of gaze producing a staring appearance; one had rapid, to-and-fro conjugate movement of the eyes.

● Twenty-two had an obviously increased and 14 an obviously decreased spontaneous blink rate; three had bursts of rapid blinking.

Exposure to neuroleptic medication did not seem to affect the presence of abnormal eye movements or blinking (see Table 8.3).

Before the introduction of neuroleptic medication in 1954, 27 had had abnormal eye movements described, including glancing away all the time, having their eyes darting to the corner of the room, gazing fixedly in random directions as if seeing things, staring up at skylights, into space or at the floor, having their eyes wandering from object to object as if they were interested or continual oscillation of the eyes; five were noted to have frequent blinking or flickering of the eyelids.

Of the 27 patients who had had abnormalities of spontaneous eye movement noted: nine were first admitted between 1907 and 1926, eight between 1927 and 1935; and 10 between 1936 and 1955. In 10, at least one of the observations was made on first admission, and in 18 within 5 years of first admission. Only 17 currently had an abnormality of spontaneous eye movement.

Abnormality of spontaneous eye movement was a feature, therefore, in a proportion of these 100 patients from fairly early on in their illness but was not necessarily a permanent feature.

Other studies

In 1978, Janice Stevens published what is still the best paper on eye movement and blinking disorders in schizophrenia (Stevens 1978a). She reported the examination of 55 patients with chronic schizophrenic illnesses who had either never received medication or had not received any for between 1 month to 4 years. Up to the time of Steven's paper, eye movement abnormalities in schizophrenia had been usually attributed to the heightened state of fear or arousal associated with acute psychosis. Their occurrence in patients with longstanding psychosis, their modulation by agents which altered central dopamine function, and the appearance of similar signs after stimulation of the mesolimbic dopaminergic system in experimental animals and during temporal lobe seizures in man led her to suggest that they represented abnormal function of the mesolimbic dopamine

Table 8.3   Percentage of patients with abnormal eye movements within various neuroleptic treatment groups

	Whole group ($n = 100$) (%)	Current ($n = 55$) (%)	Past ($n = 37$) (%)	Never ($n = 8$) (%)
Eye movements				
roving	26	27	22	38
abrupt, conjugate	28	27	30	25
Blinking				
increased	21	20	22	25
decreased	12	16	5	13

system. Karson (1979) examined the same extra-ocular movements and blink rates in 172 patients suffering from different psychiatric disorders and 32 controls, and showed that schizophrenic patients demonstrated the majority of significant deviations from the control group.

Of the 55 patients in Stevens' study, 24 had impairment of pursuit eye movements. In 1973, Holzman et al. (1973) had 're-discovered' dysfunction of smooth pursuit eye movements in patients with schizophrenia, first described at the beginning of the century. This was confirmed by several subsequent studies. Latency and velocity of visually guided saccades in such patients, however, were normal. This dissociation of smooth pursuit and saccadic eye tracking suggested that smooth-pursuit dysfunction could not be attributed to a lack of motivation, simple inattention, or oculomotor control mechanisms for which the pursuit and saccadic systems share a common anatomy (Iacono et al. 1981). Disorder of eye tracking has been reported in 51–85% of schizophrenic patients compared to 8% in controls. The abnormalities are independent of the effects of neuroleptic medication, twin and family studies have shown a high level of heritability and they can be associated with other psychiatric disorder (Blackwood et al. 1991a). The eye tracking dysfunction in schizophrenic patients is associated with enlarged cerebral ventricles and the severity of clinical symptoms, both positive and negative (Blackwood et al. 1991b).

Of the 55 patients in Stevens' study, 14 had unexplained single sustained lateral glances, which could be continuous; 12 patients had spontaneous darting, rapid, irregular searching eye movements; seven had episodes of sustained 1–2 per second horizontal oscillations of the eyes lasting 10–60 seconds. Unlike pursuit eye movement disorder, sustained spontaneous conjugate deviation of the eyes in schizophrenia has not been the subject of much interest, except as a side-effect of medication. It was the subject of a few isolated reports in the pre-neuroleptic era. Farran-Ridge (1926) described strong, upward, conjugate deviation of the eyeballs with rapid fluttering of the upper eyelids occurring in some cases of schizophrenia. Guiraud (1936) described a case of schizophrenia with stupor and hypotonia, and fixed downward spasm of the eyes persisting for over 3 months. Both these authors were interested in analogies between post-encephalitic and schizophrenic symptomatology, and drew attention to the similarity with the oculogyric crises first described after epidemic encephalitis.

However, there is very little other description in the literature of such a symptom forming part of psychiatric disorder. This is either because it was indeed uncommon or because it did occur but was included as part of the patients' abnormal mental state under the category of stereotypy or mannerism. Figure 7 supports this second possibility.

Figure 7(a) shows Guiraud's case, which appeared in his account of stereotypy, suggesting that such eye movement disorder was included in this category of movement disorder. Figure 7(b) shows the admission photograph of a patient to Friern Hospital in 1934. He was 25 years old and spent the rest of his life in Friern. His diagnosis on admission was dementia praecox and this was only changed to one of schizophrenia. His brother was a patient in Friern. He had no history of encephalitis or parkinsonism. The photograph shows upward deviation of the eyes similar to oculogyric crisis. There was no mention in his written case notes of any eye movement disorder. The only abnormality noted on neurological examination on admission to Friern was a hesitant gait. His conjugate deviation of the eyes was presumably accepted as part of his abnormal mental state.

Figure 7(c) shows a patient who was transferred to the National Hospital Queen Square in 1983 to exclude neurological disorder. He was 35 years old and had a 3-year history of depression and 6 months increasing social withdrawal and bizarre behaviour, finally becoming stuporose. He had not received neuroleptic medication. He was mute and akinetic, with flaccid tone and downward deviation of the eyes as shown. All his investigations were normal. After two treatments with electro-convulsive therapy he emerged from stupor, describing having heard the voice of his neighbour during his stupor telling him not to move, talk, eat or drink. He was returned to the referring psychiatric hospital with a diagnosis of catatonic schizophrenia. His discharge summary gave slight dehydration as his only abnormality on physical examination on admission. All his motor features, including the conjugate deviation of the eyes, were included as abnormalities of his mental state.

Once a neurological viewpoint of this motor disorder is adopted, parallels with known neurological disorders are naturally sought. Figure 7(d) shows downward oculogyric crisis following epidemic encephalitis, illustrated in Jelliffe's (1932) monograph on oculogyric crisis. This is indistinguishable from the eye movement disorder in the schizophrenic patients illustrated in Figure 7(a)–(c). In fact, post-encephalitic oculogyric crisis was a neuropsychiatric rather than a purely neurological disorder. When it was first described following encephalitis lethargica in the 1920s, the initial reaction was to consider it a hysterical phenomenon super-added to 'organic' post-encephalitic disorder (Marinesco & Radovici 1926). The deviation of the eyes could be accompanied by a wide range of psychiatric symptoms including anxiety, depression, obsessive-compulsive phenomena, ideas of reference, visual and auditory hallucinosis, delusions, and behavioural outbursts (Wimmer 1926; Jelliffe 1929; Rosner 1942).

Oculogyric crisis in patients with schizophrenia is now usually associated with neuroleptic medication, which can precipitate it as an acute dystonic reaction. Here as well, however, the motor phenomenon can be associated with psychiatric disturbance, such as auditory hallucinosis (Chiu 1989; Rogers 1989b). The association in such cases is paradoxical since an apparent side-effect of treatment is associated with a feature of the condition being treated. In the case I reported, the phenomenon had been previously noted but described as hysterical.

Sustained conjugate deviation of the eyes forms part of the motor disorder in psychiatric illness but the contribution of the disease process being treated, as opposed to the effect of treatment with neuroleptic medication, is under-recognised.

Each mammalian species has a characteristic blink rate that tends to be constant under unchanging, conditions with an inverse relationship between the rate of blinking and duration of rapid eye-movement sleep in diurnally active mammals

(Zametkin et al. 1979). This supports previous suggestions that spontaneous blinking is centrally generated and serves functions beyond simple cleansing of the eyes. Normal subjects blink at a rate of 8–22 times per minute. Spontaneous blink rates were examined during the first 2 minutes of a clinical interview in 100 psychiatric patients before the introduction of neuroleptic medication (Ostow & Ostow 1946). The 38 patients with acute psychosis, mostly schizophrenia, had a less uniform and higher blink rate (mean 27.1 per minute) than 15 recovered psychotics (mean 17.5 per minute) or the remaining patient groups.

Of the 55 patients in Stevens' study, 17 had resting blink rates in excess of 60 per minute; four patients, who had never received any medication, had blink rates of 0–1 per minute. There appears to be no method by which primary disturbance of blink regulation in schizophrenia can be reliably separated from neuroleptic-induced effects (Stevens 1978b). The mean blink rate during 3 minutes of conversation for 44 schizophrenic patients when neuroleptic medication had been withdrawn was 31 per minute, compared to 24 per minute when they were taking neuroleptic medication and 23 per minute for a group of 54 normal control subjects (Karson 1983). This lowered blink rate on neuroleptics was correlated to changes in positive symptoms and did not occur in patients with larger cerebral ventricular size on CT scan (Karson et al. 1982; Kleinman et al. 1984). Karson et al. (1990) have suggested that abnormalities of blinking in schizophrenia may be linked to the perturbed alpha rhythm on electro-encephalograms found in such patients, both representing dysfunction of a neuro-anatomical circuit linking pons, sub-cortical structures and occipital cortex. An increased mean blink rate in drug-naive schizophrenic patients and a relationship between spontaneous blink rate, positive symptomatology and neuroleptic response in schizophrenic patients has been supported by other studies (Helms & Godwin 1985; Mackert et al. 1990; Bartko et al. 1990).

Blinking rate has been studied in other psychiatric disorders. Mackintosh et al. (1983) compared the blink rates of 23 newly admitted depressed patients with that of 23 matched non-psychiatric controls. Their mean blink rate was 21.9 per minute compared to 15.2 per minute in the controls. The blink rate was lower in the depressed patients with psychomotor retardation. The depressed patients were on different medications, but the blink rate on discharge of those who improved, and who had had no significant change in medication, approached that of the controls whose blink rate remained stable on re-testing. Berrios and Canagasabey (1990) studied 28 patients with major depression before and after treatment with electroconvulsive therapy (ECT) or anti-depressant medication, which produced significant clinical improvement in some. Their mean blink rate before treatment was 21.2 blinks per minute and after treatment was 29.6 blinks per minute. Interestingly, no correlation was found between the patients' scores on Widlocher's psychomotor retardation scale and eye blink rate, either before or after treatment.

SPEECH PRODUCTION

Friern study

Of the 100 patients in the Friern study, 95 showed an abnormality of speech production.

- Twenty-two were normally mute and a further 25 only spoke occasionally.
- Fifty-three had outbursts of shouting, singing or talking lasting from a few seconds to a few days: these could be situationally provoked or apparently spontaneous and could appear on a background of mutism or reduced spontaneous speech.
- At interview, 51 produced speech so inarticulate, barely audible or even inaudible as to be unintelligible. Most of these could also produce intelligible speech but in a few, no more than isolated words or phrases. Intelligible speech could alternate with or tail off into unintelligible.

  Altogether 73 produced at least one word articulate enough to be intelligible, while 52 were able to produce more continuous, though not necessarily coherent, speech.
- In 24 of these there was an abnormality of volume, timbre or rate of delivery. The voice could be too quiet with lack of modulation, too loud, too nasal, too guttural, too slow or too fast. In one patient, as the head and trunk gradually flexed and the blink rate gradually decreased, the voice became quieter and quieter till, with the face horizontal, speech stopped altogether, resuming suddenly and loudly when the head jerked upright again, for the whole process to start again.
- Two patients had a stutter and 14 had palilalia (the repetition of the last word or phrase of a sentence). In one patient, replies to questions were preceded by three to six short grunts, building up to the explosively delivered reply, which was repeated rapidly several times. In another, replies to questions were repeated consecutively up to a dozen times, gradually becoming fainter and fainter.
- Eight had echolalia, repeating what was said to them or what they heard on television or in another conversation, which could then be incorporated into their flow of speech. Some were hardly capable of any other form of intelligible speech.
- Seven patients currently had inappropriate laughing, including a chuckle in an otherwise mute patient, and one inappropriate crying; four had respiratory tics.

Exposure to neuroleptic medication did not markedly affect the presence of speech disorder (see Table 8.4).

Table 8.4 Percentage of patients with speech disorders within various neuroleptic treatment groups

	Whole group ($n = 100$) (%)	Current ($n = 55$) (%)	Past ($n = 37$) (%)	Never ($n = 8$) (%)
Episodic vocal activity	53	60	41	63
Unintelligible speech	51	55	54	13
Mutism or no spontaneous speech	47	44	54	38
Abnormal volume, timbre or rate	24	29	16	25
Stuttering or palilalia	16	9	24	25
Echolalia	8	9	8	0

Before the first use of neuroleptic medication in the hospital in 1954, 93 patients had been noted to have a disorder of speech production:

> Altogether 62 had mutism or reduced speech production, including descriptions such as 'makes an apparently great effort to speak, when questioned, but cannot utter even a meaningless sound' or 'at times opens and closes his mouth as if speaking but without phonating'; 30, including 15 of these 62, at times showed increased or impulsive speech production with descriptions such as ' ... appears to be incapable of speech. He does, however, have sporadic impulsive talking phases which are not in response to the environment ... '; 27 had abnormalities of volume, timbre or rate of speech, with their speech described as dull, monotonous or mechanical or the voice as timid, little, thin, quiet, small, high, flat, sing-song, staccato, deep, hostile or animal like; 11 had hesitancy, stuttering or palilalia; 23 had echolalia; 38 had unintelligible speech, being noted to chatter away parrot-like, keep up an incessant babble of disconnected talk, mutter away, gabble to themselves, moan and ramble in undertones continuously, occasionally utter a stream of gibberish, shout meaningless words, have their conversation quickly degenerate into a scarcely audible mumble, make sounds in a dull monotonous manner with little apparent effort to form words, be unable to converse normally but mumble and grunt for the most part, have speech confined to inarticulate noises, snort and grunt continually during interview, whine like a dog, whinny like a mare, make an unpleasant barking sound, a loud neighing, or bird-like noises.

Of these 93 patients, in 43 one at least of the observations was noted on first admission, and in 71 within 5 years of first admission; 89 currently had disorder of speech production. Disorder of speech production, therefore, was a feature in the great majority of these 100 patients from fairly early on in their illnesses and tended to be permanent.

Altogether 41 patients had been noted to show inappropriate laughing or crying: 36 had had inappropriate laughter and 16 inappropriate crying, four being noted to alternately laugh and cry, or giggle and weep. In 27 this was first noted on first admission, and in 35 within 5 years of first admission. Only four of these currently showed inappropriate laughter or crying.

Other studies

In the Friern study, disorder of speech production mirrored disorder of the motor system generally. This has been noted by others (Manschreck 1983). There is extensive evidence that at both cortical and sub-cortical levels there is close relationship of motor and language function (Ojemann 1982).

Relatively few studies are available of specific motor speech disorders found in psychiatric patients, such as mutism and palilalia, but these show that there is a complete overlap of these disorders in psychiatric and recognised neurological disorders (Altshuler et al. 1986; Ackermann et al. 1989). Pathologic laughing and crying, a classical sign of psychiatric disorder, has likewise not been extensively studied. It is also found in patients with cerebrovascular disease or brain injury, where it is associated with decreased concentration of homovanillic acid in the cerebro-spinal fluid and to respond to treatment with levodopa or amantidine (Udaka et al. 1984).

Post-encephalitic motor disorder included speech disorder. Not one of the 130 post-encephalitic patients studied by Purdon Martin (Martin et al. 1962) had normal speech and all the speech disturbances were motor disorders of speech. None had any sign of dysphasia, five were absolutely inarticulate, some rarely spoke or were restricted to barely comprehensible whispers, and many phonated weakly or mumbled. Some could only utter isolated words fairly clearly, others after the first few words would festinate into an unintelligible jumble. This has strong parallels with the speech disorder found in the 95 patients in the Friern study described above.

The most appropriate model for the speech disorder shown by both post-encephalitic and schizophrenic patients is the concept of limbic aphasia put forward by Bryan Robinson (1976). He argued that there are two separate, parallel systems subserving speech, the limbic and the neocortical. The limbic system is bilaterally represented, has significant emotional, motivational and autonomic associations and a low information content. This is in contrast to the neocortical system, first described by Broca and Wernicke, which is lateralised, independent of emotional factors and has a high information content.

One psychiatric motor speech disorder that has been fairly extensively studied is speech pause time in depression. Szabadi et al. (1976) in fact used a technique developed for measuring periodicity of speech in parkinsonism and showed that pause time (the silent intervals between audible portions of speech) in automatic speech, such as counting, was significantly prolonged in four unmedicated depressed subjects compared to healthy subjects but this difference from controls disappeared after treatment and recovery from their depressive illness. This retardation of speech was present even when trained clinicians were unable to detect motor retardation. The association of objectively assessed speech pause time with psychomotor retardation in depressed patients and its return to normal with clinical improvement was confirmed by subsequent studies (Teasdale et al. 1980; Greden et al. 1981; Godfrey & Knight 1984; Hardy et al. 1984; Hoffmann et al. 1985), although not all studies (Nilsonne 1988). Widlocher's group (Hardy et al. 1984) and Hoffman's showed a strong correlation between this speech pause time and Widlocher's depressive retardation rating scale, as well as simple reaction time. These findings prompted Greden and Carroll (1981) to suggest that the speech disturbance in depressive illness was due to the same dysfunction of meso-limbic/nigro-striatal dopamine projection systems which had been demonstrated in Parkinson's disease.

Conclusion

To have forgotten that schizophrenia is a brain disease will go down as one of the great aberrations of twentieth century medicine (Ron & Harvey 1990).

It is only a matter of time before similar statements are made about other psychiatric disorders. There are not two types of psychiatric disorder, but two ways of looking at psychiatric disorder. There is not brain-based psychiatric disorder and non-brain-based disorder, but a brain-based and a non-brain-based approach to understanding psychiatric disorder. Both approaches are equally valid. The appropriate approach is the one that makes most sense of a particular disorder and leads to effective treatment.

The foundations for a brain-based approach to understanding psychiatric disorder were laid down at the end of the last century, but an alternative way of making sense of psychiatric disorder, a non-brain-based psychological approach, has dominated twentieth-century psychiatry. Over the last 25 years a 'silent' revolution has been taking place in psychiatry, as a brain-based approach has gradually been gaining ground again. One could say that psychiatry has finally moved into the twentieth century in time for the start of the twenty-first.

We still have some way to go, however, to reach the position where Griesinger and Maudsley left off. Of over 15 000 psychiatric articles published in the period 1981–85, over two-thirds fell into the category of psychosocial psychiatry with only a quarter dealing with the objective, biological, cognitive, neuroscientific aspects of psychiatry (Wortis 1990). Research findings increasingly demonstrate a high prevalence of abnormal neurological findings in patients having valid primary psychiatric diagnoses, but clinical psychiatric practice continues to limit the role for neurology in psychiatry to the screening of psychiatric patients for the presence of unsuspected neurological disease (Woods & Short 1985).

Every psychiatrist examines motor function in his patients every time he sees them and this forms an important part of their assessment of mental state and diagnosis. With a neurological perspective of psychiatric disorder, this assessment is examination of the nervous system. With a brain-based approach, physical symptoms of psychiatric disorder are of equal interest to the mental symptoms and the clinical overlap of psychiatric disorder and recognised neurological disorder becomes of immediate interest. The present book is an exploration of the suggestion that motor disorder forms a significant part of psychiatric disorder, and that there is a significant overlap between this motor disorder and motor disorder associated with accepted neurological disorders.

There is currently a considerable research effort in both psychiatry and neurology which overlaps but paradoxically does not meet. For example, a significant divide is made between the mesolimbic and nigrostriatal dopamine projection systems from brainstem to forebrain, with the former designated as psychiatric and the latter as neurological territory. Topographical studies, however, have consistently shown that the dopamine neurons of the substantia nigra-ventral tegmental area form a single nuclear group and that these meso-telencephalic neurons should be regarded as a single system with a lateral to medial topographic arrangement in their projections to striatal and limbic cortical areas (Fallon & Moore 1978; Bjorklund & Lindvall 1978).

There is not a 'psychiatric brain' and a 'neurological brain'. There is only one brain. Psychiatric disorder represents valuable data for the understanding of normal and abnormal brain functioning. Simply bringing together research efforts in neurology and psychiatry could achieve a quantum leap of understanding of psychiatric disorder and cerebral function.

Rating Scales for Motor Disorder in Psychiatry

Standardised rating scales for motor disorder are a fairly recent development. They appeared first for neurological disorder but, by and large, psychiatrists have been more assiduous in the development of standardised rating scales. The following four scales are useful in the assessment of motor disorder in psychiatric patients. This is currently mainly in a research setting, either for disease-based disorder or assessment of treatment, but could be incorporated into clinical assessments as a neurological perspective of psychiatric disorder develops.

WEBSTER RATING SCALE FOR PARKINSONISM (WEBSTER 1968)

This is one of the standard neurological rating scales used for assessing the severity of Parkinson's disease. It has also been used in patients with primary depressive illness (Rogers et al. 1987) and schizophrenic illness (McKenna et al. 1991).

1. *Bradykinesia of hands*
   0—no involvement
   1—detectable slowness
   2—moderate slowness
   3—severe slowness. Unable to write or button clothes
2. *Rigidity*
   0—none detectable
   1—mild rigidity detectable only on activation
   2—moderate rigidity detectable at rest
   3—severe resting rigidity
3. *Posture*
   0—normal posture; head flexed forward less than 4 inches
   1—beginning poker spine; head flexed forwards
   2—one or both arms flexed but still below waist
   3—simian posture
4. *Upper extremity swing*
   0—both arms swing well
   1—one arm definitely decreased in amount of swing
   2—one arm fails to swing
   3—both arms fail to swing

5. *Gait*

    0—steps out well with 18–30 inch stride

    1—stride 12–18 inches; strikes one heel; takes several steps to turn

    2—stride 6–12 inches; both heels strike floor forcefully

    3—shuffling gait and/or propulsion and intermittent freezing

6. *Tremor*

    0—no detectable tremor

    1—mild fine-amplitude tremor; may be asymptomatic

    2—severe but not constant; patient retains control of hands

    3—constant and severe; writing and feeding are impossible

7. *Facies*

    0—normal; full animation; no stare

    1—detectable immobility

    2—moderate immobility; drooling may be present

    3—frozen facies; mouth open; drooling may be severe

8. *Seborrhoea*

    0—none

    1—increased perspiration; secretion remains thin

    2—obvious oiliness; secretion much thicker

    3—marked seborrhoea; entire face and head covered by thick secretion

9. *Speech*

    0—clear, loud, resonant, easily understood

    1—beginning of hoarseness with loss of inflection and resonance; good volume and still easily understood

    2—moderate hoarseness and weakness; beginning of dysarthria, hesitancy, stuttering, difficult to understand

    3—marked harshness and weakness; very difficult to hear and understand

10. *Self-care*

    0—no impairment

    1—still provides full self-care but rate of dressing impeded

    2—requires help in certain critical areas, such as turning in bed, rising from chairs, etc.; very slow in performing most activities but manages by taking much time

    3—continuously disabled; unable to dress, feed himself, or walk alone

ABNORMAL INVOLUNTARY MOVEMENT SCALE (AIMS)
(Guy 1976)

This has mainly been used in the assessment of drug-related tardive dyskinesia but there is no reason why it could not be used to assess dyskinesia of any cause. The scale has 12 items. The highest severity of abnormal movements observed in each of seven body parts should be rated, with movements occurring on activation being rated one less than those observed spontaneously. The first seven items are rated:

0—none
1—minimal, may be extreme normal
2—mild
3—moderate
4—severe

1. *Muscles of facial expression*
   For example, movements of forehead, eyebrows, peri-orbital area, cheeks; include frowning, blinking, smiling, grimacing.
2. *Lips and peri-oral area*
   For example, puckering, pouting, smacking.
3. *Jaw*
   For example, biting, clenching, chewing, mouth opening, lateral movements.
4. *Tongue*
   Only increase in movement both in and out of mouth, not inability to sustain movement.
5. *Upper extremity movements*
   (Arms, wrists, hands, fingers) including choreic (i.e. rapid, objectively purposeless, irregular, spontaneous) and athetoid (i.e. slow, irregular, complex, serpentine) movements but not tremor (i.e. repetitive, regular, rhythmic).
6. *Lower extremity movements*
   (Legs, knees, ankles, toes) e.g. lateral knee movement, foot tapping, heel dropping, foot squirming, inversion and eversion of foot.
7. *Neck, shoulders, hips*
   For example, rocking, twisting, squirming, pelvic gyrations.

The next two items are global items rated in the same fashion:

8. *Global severity of abnormal movements*
9. *Incapacitation due to abnormal movements*

The next item is rated:

0—no awareness
1—aware, no distress
2—aware, mild distress
3—aware, moderate distress
4—aware, severe distress

10. *Patient's awareness of abnormal movements*
    (i.e. patient's report)

The last two items are rated no/yes:

11. *Current problems with teeth and/or dentures*
12. *Does patient usually wear dentures?*

DEPRESSIVE RETARDATION RATING SCALE (Widlocher 1983)[*]

This was developed, after two preliminary versions, by Widlocher and his colleagues at the Salpetriere Hospital in Paris. The scale was tested on two groups of depressed patients: 142 in-patients and 84 out-patients. It measures a single dimension accounting for nearly 60% of the variance, and there is a close correlation of almost all the items within this factor. The total score discriminates depressed patients from normal subjects. In depressed patients it is usually well above 20, while in normal subjects it is usually under 16. This total score correlates significantly with global rating on the Hamilton Depression Rating Scale (Hamilton 1960), and especially the retardation item on this scale, both on single measurements at one point in time and repeated measures on the same patients, with high inter-rater correlation of scores on different items (Jouvent et al. 1980).

The scale has 15 items: three items assess motor function, three speech production, two objective mental activity and six subjective experience with a further item for overall assessment. Each item is scored on a 0–4 scale:

Motor function
1. *Gait*
   0—normal
   1—mild slowing but of uncertain pathological significance
   2—one of the following is observed
      (a) a lack of suppleness of stride or arm swing
      (b) dragging of the feet
      (c) slow stride of normal amplitude
      (d) slow small-stepped stride
   3—more than one of the features in 2 (above)
   4—cannot walk without support
2. *Movement of trunk and limbs*
   0—appropriate movements of normal amplitude, suppleness and rhythmicity; comfortable sitting posture with relaxed shoulders; posture and movements in harmony with conversation
   1—mild cramping of movements, barely noticeable
   2—lack of associated movement definitely present
   3—limbs moved only rarely, and then more slowly than usual with awkwardness of gesture and reduced amplitude of movement or fixity of proximal portions of arms with only the hands moving; immobile trunk, either plastered against back of chair or with drooping of shoulders

---

[*] Reproduced by permission of W. B. Saunders Co.

4—refuses to get out of bed or immobile in chair; complete absence of truncal movements and complete lack of associated movement

3. *Movement of face, head and neck*

    0—free movements of head, independent of body movements, the gaze either exploring the room or fixed on the examiner or objects of interest in an appropriate fashion; normal amplitude of mouth movements

    1—some reduction of mobility, not necessarily persistent

    2—mild but definite reduced mobility; gaze often fixed but capable of shifting; monotonous quality to facial movements, though some expressiveness possible

    3—no head movements; no visual exploration of room and usually staring at floor, seldom looking at examiner; poor articulation, hardly moving the mouth; no smiling, unchanging expression

    4—face completely immobile and painfully inexpressive

Speech production

4. *Flow of speech*

    0—normal

    1—hardly perceptible slowing of speech

    2—definite slowing of speech not interfering with conversation

    3—any speech requires forceful urging by examiner

    4—stereotyped responses

5. *Voice*

    0—normal

    1—hardly perceptible reduction of volume

    2—reduced volume and monotonous—listener must lean closer

    3—voice hardly audible—listener must ask for certain phrases to be repeated

    4—inaudible speech

6. *Verbal responses*

    0—no difficulty making responses of appropriate length

    1—responses somewhat briefer than expected

    2—brief responses but not interfering with course of conversation

    3—responses restricted to just a few words

    4—only monosyllabic replies

Objective mental activity

7. *Spontaneous speech*

    0—variety of themes broached by subject, smooth transition from one theme to another

    1—conversational themes relatively varied but some difficulty making quick transition from one subject to another

    2—reduced number of new themes and not fully developed

    3—no spontaneous new themes with a tendency to ruminate on certain ideas

    4—conversation meagre, monotonous, exploration of new themes resisted

8. *Elicited speech*

0—easy and ready associations to conversational themes proposed

1—themes developed fairly readily but some difficulty moving from one theme to the next

2—themes rarely developed and showing little variety

3—no new themes developed, tendency to rumination

4—extremely meagre conversation

Subjective experience

9. *Ruminations*

0—no impairment of thought

1—possible impairment approaching 2

2—thoughts tend to dwell on two or three themes that recur over and over again, impairing functioning

3—thoughts always return to single painful preoccupation

4—total incapacity to escape from painful preoccupations

10. *Fatiguability*

0—none mentioned spontaneously or on direct questioning

1—not mentioned spontaneously but evidence of fatiguability emerges during course of interview

2—distress due to fatiguability in activities of daily living

3—fatiguability leads to reduced activity

4—almost complete reduction of activity due to overwhelming fatigue

11. *Interest in normal activities*

0—usual interests retained despite hospitalisation or treatment

1—some loss of interest ascribed to hospitalisation or other pretext

2—cessation of certain activities due to loss of interest

3—extensive loss of interest, including subject's future

4—complete loss of interest

12. *Time perception*

0—same as usual

1—time seems to pass slowly due to inactivity or being in hospital, etc.

2—passage of time seems slower on direct questioning

3—slowing of passage of time mentioned spontaneously or quite readily on direct questioning

4—passage of time seems suspended; painful perception of an 'infinite present'

13. *Memory*

0—no difficulty subjectively or in conversation

1—some subjective difficulty but not apparent in conversation

2—apparent difficulty in conversation but no handicap to subject

3—memory difficulty a handicap

4—significant amnesia

14. *Concentration*
    0—normal
    1—subjectively normal, but certain tasks requiring concentration seem difficult
    2—difficulty with certain tasks such as reading, calculation and professional tasks
    3—serious difficulty interfering with ordinary activities, such as reading newspaper, watching television, etc.
    4—difficulty concentrating during interview

Overall assessment
15. *Psychomotor retardation*
    0—none
    1—equivocal
    2—mild but definite
    3—moderate
    4—severe

CATATONIA—THE MODIFIED ROGERS SCALE (Lund et al. 1991)[*]

This rates both extrapyramidal and catatonic abnormalities, as well as those potentially classifiable as either, in patients with schizophrenia. As well as removing the need to try and decide this at the time of rating, this non-prejudicial approach permits a score to be derived for catatonic symptoms 'uncontaminated' by phenomena currently accepted as extrapyramidal.

Items on the scale identified as potentially extrapyramidal include those characteristic of parkinsonism or involuntary movement disorders and those explicitly or implicitly associated with extrapyramidal syndromes.

The remaining items can be considered as a subscale rating, phenomena falling outside the normal range of neuroleptic-induced parkinsonism and dyskinesia, approximating fairly closely to classically described catatonic symptoms.

The scale is easy to use and most patients are able to comply with the examination. Even when this is not the case, many items can be completed by observation or questioning of nursing staff. It is the only currently available rating scale for catatonia.

The reliability and validity of the scale was determined by examination of 93 acute and chronic schizophrenic in-patients using two pairs of independent raters. A number of patients were re-examined 1–6 months after their original assessment. The same patients were also rated with the Behavioural Observation Schedule (BOS) (Atakan and Cooper 1989) and Social Behavioural Schedule (SBS) (Wykes and Sturt 1986).

---

[*] Reproduced by permission of the Royal College of Psychiatrists.

The Modified Rogers Scale (MRS) is reliable. Most items show high inter-rater reliability and test–re-test scores were not significantly different. Total scores on the MRS were highly significantly correlated with total BOS scores and the highest correlation of all was between total scores on the MRS and summed scores on individual BOS items rating specific motor, volitional and behavioural disorder. Total scores on the MRS were also highly significantly correlated with nurses' ratings on the motor, volitional and behavioural subset of the SBS. For the catatonic subscale of the MRS, six category subscale scores were on the whole inter correlated with each other and each of the six was highly significantly correlated with the total catatonic score.

All abnormalities are rated phenomenologically, regardless of their presumed basis (i.e. extrapyramidal or catatonic). Abnormalities that are questionable, subtle or only minimally present should not be rated.

There are 36 items each rated:

0—abnormality absent
1—abnormality definitely present
2—abnormality marked or pervasive

The 36 items are grouped into 10 categories:

Posture
  1. *Simple abnormal posture*
     Generally relatively fixed; specify: flexed, lordotic, twisted, tilted, other.
  2. *Complex abnormal posture*
     May be more dynamic, e.g. slack, constrained, awkward; 'posturing'—2.
  3. *Persistence of imposed postures*
     Not sustained—1, sustained 'waxy flexibility'—2.

Tone and motor compliance
  4. *Abnormal tone*
     Specify: increased, decreased.
  5. *Gegenhalten*
     'Springy' resistance to passive movement, which increases with increasing force.
  6. *Mitgehen*
     'Anglepoise lamp' raising of arm in response to light pressure; do not rate if poor understanding of instruction.

Abnormal movements: face and head
  7. *Simple brief/dyskinesia-like*
     Specify: random/irregularly, repetitive/rhythmical/tic-like.
  8. *Simple sustained/grimace-like*
     For example, spasmodic facial contortions; should not be completely fixed.
  9. *Complex mannerism/stereotypy-like*
     Usually of head, e.g. turning away, side-to-side looks, searching movements.

Abnormal movements: trunk and limbs
10. *Simple brief/dyskinesia-like*
    Specify: random/irregularly, repetitive/rhythmical/tic-like; include rocking
11. *Simple sustained/dystonia-like*
    For example, dystonic posturing of extremities, hyperpronation on arm raising, torsion movements.
12. *Complex mannerisms/stereotypy-like*
    For example, touching, stroking, finger play, repetitious gestures.

Abnormal ocular movements
13. *Increased blinking*
    Including rapid bursts.
14. *Decreased blinking*
15. *Eye movements*
    Specify: to-and-fro/roving/conjugate deviation.

Purposive movement
16. *Abruptness/rapidity of spontaneous movements*
    For example, sudden gestures, acts carried out smartly, springs to attention when asked to stand.
17. *Slowness/feebleness of spontaneous movements*
    For example, weak, languid, laboured.
18. *Exaggerated quality to movements*
    Accompanied by flourishes/flurries of adventitious movements—2.
19. *Iterations of spontaneous movements*
    For example, gesture/mannerism repeated.
20. *Other*
    Specify: echopraxia/blocking/ambitendence; do not rate any other abnormalities than these.

Gait
21. *Exaggerated associated movement*
    Rate irrespective of 24.
22. *Reduced associated movement*
    Rate irrespective of 24.
23. *Slow/shuffling*
24. *Manneristic/bizarre*
    May be extravagant or constrained quality or neither; do not rate merely clumsy, hunched or lordotic gaits; interpolated movements—2.

Speech
25. *Aprosodic*
    Markedly abnormal rate/volume/intonation, e.g. rasping, sing-song, automaton-like; do not rate mere lack of inflection.
26. *Mutism*
    Less than 20 words—1, no speech—2.

27. *Indistinct/unintelligible speech*
   For example, mumbling/poor, articulation/non-social speech; verbigeration —2.
28. *Other*
   Specify: echolalia/palilalia/speech mannerism; do not rate any other abnormalities than these.

Behaviour during interview

29. *Marked overactivity*
   1—in constant motion/continual succession of mannerisms and stereotypies;
   2—approaching catatonic excitement; do not rate simple restlessness/ akathisia; do not rate unless substantial.
30. *Marked underactivity*
   1—sits abnormally still, inert, passive; 2—approaching stupor; do not rate if patient is clearly sedated/parkinsonian; do not rate unless substantial.
31. *Excessive compliance/automatic obedience*
   For example, raises both arms when asked to raise one, continues to carry out instructed actions unnecessarily, obeys instructions instantly.
32. *Poor/feeble compliance*
   Failure to perform, carry through or maintain requested actions not due to general unco-operativeness or poor understanding; do not rate if clearly parkinsonian.
33. *Other*
   Specify: negativism/hypermetamorphosis; do not rate any other abnormalities but these.

Reported behaviour

34. *Overactive*
   For example, restless, paces, wanders all day.
35. *Underactive*
   For example, sits in same place all day, has to be brought to the meal table.
36. *Other*
   For example, adopts postures, performs repetitive acts, engages in rituals.

Guidelines for rating catatonic phenomena

Complex abnormal posture

Mere ungainliness or slouching should not be rated.

Rating 1

For example: assuming obviously abnormal hunched, constrained, 'closed' or alternatively exaggeratedly slack, over-relaxed positions when sitting; hugging sides, twisting legs round each other, sitting with torso forward but legs to one side in extremely uncomfortable way.

Rating 2
For example: while sitting, repeatedly hunching forward and rocking; while standing or walking, striking a series of poses.

Persistence of imposed postures

Rating 1
For example, tendency to retain limb positions passively imposed during testing for at least several seconds; this should be observed more than once.

Rating 2
For example, typical waxy flexibility.

Gegenhalten

Resistance to passive movement, which increases with the force exerted; typically has a 'springy' quality and appears automatic rather than wilful. May be restricted to just one muscle group, e.g. the neck.

Mitgehen

'Anglepoise lamp' arm raising in response to light pressure, in the presence of an apparent grasp of the need to resist; should be demonstrable repeatedly. Severity of rating depends on the rapidity and apparent wish to anticipate the movement; other similar tests, such as tipping the patient backwards by lightly pressing on the forehead or turning him/her round by light pressure on an outstretched arm, can also be used.

Complex sterotypy/mannerism-like movements

More stereotypy-like examples are: rubbing the thumb over the forefinger, other kinds of finger play, touching, rubbing, stroking and patting various parts of the body especially the face, and repeatedly turning the head away from the examiner, looking round distractedly throughout the interview, twisting one arm up behind the back while walking, repeatedly rising from chair and approaching examiner. More mannerism-like examples are holding arms in an unnatural crooked way, holding an arm out in a meaningless gesture, keeping one arm tucked under armpit.

Iterations

Gestures or mannerisms repeated over short space of time, e.g. touching face then repeating this several times; manneristically smoothing hair, then repeating this with increasing force until striking head; touching ring finger on one hand (while alluding to ring being stolen), then doing the same on the other hand, then repeating the whole sequence.

Echopraxia

Incomplete copying movements should not be rated, and exercise judgement as to whether patient is just trying to be helpful. As well as being merely copied, movements may be modified or amplified, e.g., smoothing of hair substituted for examiner's scratching of head, echopraxic chest patting progressively exaggerated until patient is pulling at his shirt.

Blocking/ambitendence

In practice not easy to distinguish from one another. Examples are: freezing in the act of sitting forward and remaining motionless, grasping the arms of the chair for nearly a minute; extending arm when examiner's is proffered, then halting in mid-action and moving arm to one side; while walking, stopping, half-turning back, then continuing.

Manneristic/bizarre gait

Merely clumsy or lumbering gaits should not be rated, and gait should be idiosyncratic rather than hunched, lordotic, shuffling, etc. Examples are: constrained, mincing, over-precise; or alternatively extravagant, over-elaborate, featuring interpolated movements, such as sidesteps and bowing, and also bizarre crab-like, crouching or anthropoid gaits, and those with multiple, not easily described abnormalities.

Aprosodic speech

Simply unvarying, harsh or stereotyped inflections should not be rated unless marked. Examples are: unnaturally loud, strident, high-pitched; or alternatively feeble, whispering or completely monotonous intonations. Occasionally also automaton-like, sing-song, rasping, strangled, or warbling inflections.

Overactivity/excitement

Typically bizarre rather than resembling simple restlessness; akathisia should be excluded where suspected.

Rating 1
Continual motor unrest. For example; crossing and uncrossing legs, looking round, half rising from the chair; executing unending series of manneristic actions, touching body, then clasping hands, then gripping the chair arm, etc.

Rating 2

In more or less constant motion, incessantly performing pointless actions which are reiterated, elaborated and transformed into one another, for example, touching cardigan, then moving hands up and down the edges, then unbuttoning it and buttoning it up again, followed by breaking off interview to clamber over the tables and chairs on the ward. Also includes full-blown excitement, for example, a patient who moves round and round the ward striking an endless series of quasi-symbolic poses.

Underactivity/stupor

Some degree of abnormality is commonly observed and should not be rated unless very noticeable.

Rating 1

Sitting abnormally still throughout the interview with hardly any postural shifts; slumped in chair; very passive.

Rating 2

Marked hypokinesia, generally with striking absence of postural adjustments, for example, sitting perched on chair in same position throughout interview, not turning head when addressed from different direction; always sitting in same place on ward with arms held in praying position. Also includes full blown stupor if encountered.

Excessive compliance/automatic obedience

May take the form of exaggerated co-operation with instructed movements, for example, when asked to lift a finger, whole arm raised; when asked to lower arm, done so smartly that it overshoots backwards; when arm reached for, whole body leant forward and turned towards examiner; holding out both hands when examiner's offered for shaking. Alternatively, spontaneous continuation of actions, for example, flapping arms when asked to drop them to sides, actively continuing passive arm movements during examination for tone; occasionally, complying with all requests to an extraordinary degree, for example, screwing up eyes when asked to look out of window; when asked to keep head up while walking, proceeding across the room with neck hyperextended.

Poor/feeble compliance

Inability to perform requested actions not explicable in terms of poor understanding, general unco-operativeness, blocking/ambitendence, or parkinsonism; often has a bizarre quality. Examples are: when raising arm, movement gradually dies away; carries out most instructions promptly but fails to comply with some;

seems unable to maintain arms outstretched; when asked to hold out arms only seems able to do so in half-hearted, crooked way; when asked to raise a finger, after some delay lifts thumb.

Negativism

Should always reflect concrete instances rather than indefinable attitude. Examples are: pulling arm violently away whenever the examiner reaches for it, holding breath when asked to breathe deeply, shutting eyes tightly when approached with an ophthalmoscope, jumping up when asked to lie down, taking off socks when told to put shoes on; getting up from customary reclining position and walking away whenever approached by examiner; occasionally, domination of entire behaviour by bizarre contrariness, for example, a normally quiet patient who meets attempts to examine him with immediate struggling and vilification; leaning backwards when pulled forwards; refusing to stand up, then refusing to sit down again.

Hypermetamorphosis

Typically only seen in setting of marked overactivity, for example, attention repeatedly drawn by specks, bits of fluff, etc., on the floor, which are reached for and scrutinised; randomly approaching various objects including wastebasket, rummaging in it, extracting apple core and eating it.

References

Arahamson I. & Rabiner A.N. (1924) Some phasic and permanent mutations in certain encephalitic syndromes. *Journal of Nervous and Mental Diseases*, **60**, 249–61.

Abrams R. & Taylor M.A. (1976) Catatonia, a prospective clinical study. *Archives of General Psychiatry*, **33**, 579–81.

Achte K.A. (1961) The course of schizophrenic and schizophreniform psychoses. *Acta Psychiatrica et Neurologica Scandinavica*, **36** (suppl. 155), 220–7.

Ackermann H., Ziegler W. & Oertel W.H. (1989) Palilalia as a symptom of levodopa induced hyperkinesia in Parkinson's disease. *Journal of Neurology, Neurosurgery and Psychiatry*, **52**, 805–7.

Adland M.L. (1947) Review, case studies, therapy, and interpretation of the acute exhaustive psychoses. *Psychiatric Quarterly*, **21**, 38–69.

Agid Y., Ruberg M., Dubois B. & Javoy-Agid F. (1984) Biochemical substrates of mental disturbances in Parkinson's disease. In: R. G. Hassler & J.F. Christ (Eds.), *Advances in Neurology*, Vol. 40, pp. 211–8. Raven Press: New York.

Ajuriaguerra J. de (1971a) Étude psychopathologique des Parkinsoniens. In: J. de Ajuriaguerra & G. Gauthier (Eds.), *Monoamines, Noyaux Gris Centraux et Syndrome de Parkinson*, pp. 327–51. Georg: Geneva.

Ajuriaguerra J. de (1975) The concept of akinesia. *Psychological Medicine*, **5**, 129–37.

Albert M.L., Feldman R.G. & Willis A.L. (1974) The 'subcortical dementia' of progressive supranuclear palsy. *Journal of Neurology, Neurosurgery and Psychiatry*, **37**, 121–30.

Alexander G.E. (1986) Parallel organization of functionally segregated circuits linking basal ganglia and cortex. *Annual Review of Neurosciences*, **9**, 357–81.

Altshuler L.L., Cummings J.L. & Mills M.J. (1986) Mutism: review, differential diagnosis, and report of 22 cases. *American Journal of Psychiatry*, **143**, 1409–14.

Anderson C.M. (1952) Organic factors predisposing to schizophrenia. *The Nervous Child*, **10**, 36–42.

Andreasen N.C. (1989a) Scale for the assessment of negative symptoms (SANS) *British Journal of Psychiatry*, **155** (suppl. 7), 53–8.

Andreasen N.C. (1989b) Neural mechanisms of negative symptoms. *British Journal of Psychiatry*, **155** (suppl. 7), 93–8.

Arieti S. (1945) Primitive habits and perceptual alterations in terminal stage of schizophrenia. *Archives of Neurology and Psychiatry*, **53**, 378–84.

Arieti S. (1959)   Schizophrenia: the manifest symptomatology, the psycho-
   dynamic and formal mechanisms. In: S. Arieti, (Ed.), *American Handbook of
   Psychiatry*, Vol. 1, pp. 455–84. New York: Basic Books Inc.
Arieti S. (1972)   Volition and value: a study based on catatonic schizophrenia.
   In: S.C. Post (Ed.), *Moral Values and the Superego Concept in Psychoanalysis*,
   pp. 275–88. International Universities Press: New York.
Aring C.D. (1962)   The riddle of the Parkinson syndrome. *Archives of Neuro-
   logy*, 6, 1–4.
Armon, C. (1991)   The alternating eye deviation sign. *Neurology*, 41, 1845.
Atakan Z. & Cooper J.E. (1989)   Behavioural Observation Schedule (BOS), PIRS
   2nd edition. *British Journal of Psychiatry*, 155 (suppl. 7), 78–88.
Azima H. & Sarwer-Foner G.J. (1960)   Psychoanalytic formulations the effect of
   drugs in pharmacotherapy. *Revue Canadienne de Biologie*, 20, 425–49.
Babcock H. (1933)   *Dementia Praecox: a Psychological Study*. Science Press: New
   York.
Ball B. (1882)   De l'insanite dans la paralysie agitante. *l'Encephale*, 2, 22–32.
Banki C.M. (1977)   Correlation between cerebrospinal fluid amine metabolites
   and psychomotor activity in affective disorders. *Journal of Neurochemistry*, 28,
   255–7.
Barnes T.E. & Bridges P.K. (1980)   Disturbed behaviour induced by high-dose
   antipsychotic drugs. *British Medical Journal*, 285, 274–5.
Barnes M.P., Saunders M., Walls T.J., Saunders I. & Kirk C.A. (1986)   The
   syndrome of Karl Ludwig Kahlbaum. *Journal of Neurology, Neurosurgery and
   Psychiatry*, 49, 991–6.
Bartko G., Herczeg I. & Zador G. (1990)   Blink rate response to haloperidol as
   possible predictor of therapeutic outcome. *Biological Psychiatry*, 27, 113–5.
Barton R. (1976)   *Institutional Neurosis*, 3rd edn. John Wright: Bristol.
Baumeister A.A., MacLean W.E., Kelly J. & Casari C. (1980)   Observational
   studies of retarded children with multiple stereotyped movements. *Journal of
   Abnormal Child Psychology*, 8, 501–21.
Bergen J.A., Eyland E.A., Campbell J.A., Jenkins P., Kelleher K., Richards A.
   & Beaumont P.J.V. (1989)   The course of tardive dyskinesia in patients on
   long-term neuroleptics. *British Journal pf Psychiatry*, 154, 523–8.
Berlin L. (1955)   Compulsive eye opening and associated phenomena. *Archives
   of Neurology and Psychiatry*, 73, 597–601.
Berrios G.E. (1981)   Stupor: a conceptual history. *Psychological Medicine*, 11,
   677–88.
Berrios G.E. & Canagasabey A.F.B. (1990)   Depression, eye blink rate, psycho-
   motor retardation, and electroconvulsive therapy enhanced dopamine receptor
   sensitivity. *Convulsive Therapy*, 6, 224–30.
Bhugra D. & Baker S. (1990)   State-dependent tardive dyskinesia. *Journal of
   Nervous and Mental Disease*, 178, 720.
Bishop M.P., Gallant D.M. & Sykes T.F. (1965)   Extrapyramidal side effects and
   therapeutic response. *Archives of General Psychiatry*, 13, 155–62.

Bjorklund A. & Lindvall O. (1978) The meso-telencephalic dopamine neuron system: a review of its anatomy. In: K.E. Livingston & O. Hornykiewicz (Eds.), *Limbic Mechanisms: the Continuing Evolution of the Limbic System Concept*, pp. 307–31. Plenum Press: New York.

Blackwood D.H.R., St Clair D.M., Muir W.J. & Duffy J.C. (1991a) Auditory P300 and eye tracking dysfunction in schizophrenic pedigrees. *Archives of General Psychiatry*, **48**, 899–909.

Blackwood D.H.R., Young A.H., McQueen J.K., Martin M.J., Roxborough H.M., Muir W.J., St Clair D.M. & Kean D.M. (1991b) Magnetic resonance imaging in schizophrenia: altered brain morphology associated with P300 abnormalities and eye tracking dysfunction. *Biological Psychiatry*, **30**, 753–69.

Bleuler E. (1911) *Dementia Praecox Oder die Gruppe der Schophrenien*. Deuticke: Liepzig.

Bleuler E. (1923) *Textbook of Psychiatry*, translated by A.A. Brill. George Allen & Unwin: London.

Bleuler E. (1930) The physiogenic and psychogenic in schizophrenia. *American Journal of Psychiatry*, **110**, 203–11.

Brand N. & Jolles J. (1987) Information processing in depression anxiety. *Psychological Medicine*, **17**, 145–53.

Brandon S., McClelland H.A. & Protheroe C. (1971) A study of facial dyskinesia in a mental hospital population. *British Journal of Psychiatry*, **118**, 171–84.

Brenner C., Friedman A.P. & Merritt H.H. (1947) Psychiatric syndromes in patients with organic brain disease. 1. Diseases of the basal ganglia. *American Journal of Psychiatry*, **103**, 733–7.

Brenner I. & Rheuban W.J. (1978) The catatonic dilemma. *American Journal of Psychiatry*, **135**, 1242–3.

Brickner, R.M., Rosner, A.A. & Monro R. (1940) Physiological aspects of the obessive state. *Psychosomatic Medicine*, **2**, 369–83.

Brooks, G.W. (1956) Experience with the use of chlorpromazine and reserpine in psychiatry with especial reference to the significance and management of extrapyramidal dysfunction. *New England Journal of Medicine*, **254**, 1119–23.

Cairns H., Oldfield R.C., Pennybacker J.B. & Whitteridge D. (1941) Akinetic mutism with an epidermoid cyst of the third ventricle. *Brain*, **64**, 273–90.

Cairns H. (1952) Disturbances of consciousness with lesions of the brain-stem and diencephalon. *Brain*, **75**, 109–46.

Carluccio C., Sours J.A. & Kolb L.C. (1964) Psychodynamics of echo-reactions. *Archives of General Psychiatry*, **10**, 623–9.

Chapman J. (1966) The early symptoms of schizophrenia. *British Journal of Psychiatry*, **112**, 225–51.

Chapman J. & McGhie A. (1964) Echopraxia in schizophrenia. *British Journal of Psychiatry*, **110**, 365–74.

Chia L-G. (1991) Locked-in syndrome with bilateral ventral midbrain infarcts. *Neurology*, **41**, 445–6.

Chiu L.P.W. (1989) Transient recurrence of auditory hallucinations during acute dystonia. *British Journal of Psychiatry*, **155**, 110–13.

Chorfi M. & Moussaoui D. (1985) Les schizophrenes jamais traites n'ont pas de mouvements anormaux type dyskinesie tardive. *L'Encephale*, **XI**, 263–5.

Clarke D.J. & Brown N.S. (1990) Kluver–Bucy syndrome and psychiatric illness. *British Journal of Psychiatry*, **157**, 439–41.

Claude H., Baruk H. & Lamanche A. (1927a) Obsessions compulsions consecutive a l'encephalite epidemique. *Encephale*, **22**, 716.

Claude H., Baruk H. & Thevenard A. (1927b) Le syndrome moteur de la demence precoce catatonique. *Encephale*, **22**, 741–67.

Claude H. & Baruk H. (1928) Les crises de catalepsie. Leur diagnostic avec le sommeil pathologique. Leers rapports avec l'hysterie et la catatonie. *Encephale*, **23**, 373–402.

Cornell D.G., Suarez R. & Berent S. (1984) Psychomotor retardation in melancholic and nonmelancholic depression: cognitive and motor components. *Journal of Abnormal Psychology*, **93**, 150–7.

Court J.H. (1964) A longitudinal study of psychomotor functioning in acute psychiatric patients. *British Journal of Medical Psychology*, **37**, 167–73.

Crane G.E. (1973) Persistent dyskinesia. *British Journal of Psychiatry*, **122**, 395–405.

Critchley M. (1964) The neurology of psychotic speech. *British Journal of Psychiatry*, **110**, 353–64.

Crow T.J., Cross A.J., Johnstone E.C., Owen F., Owens D.G.C. & Waddington J.L. (1982) Abnormal involuntary movements in schizophrenia: are they related to the disease process or its treatment? Are they associated with changes in dopamine receptors? *Journal of Clinical Psychopharmacology*, **2**, 336–40.

Cruchet R. (1921) La forme bradykinesique (ou pseudo-parkinsonienne) de l'encephalomyelite epidemique. *Revue Neurologique*, **28**, 665–72.

Cummings J.L. & Frankel M. (1985) Gilles de la Tourette syndrome and the neurological basis of obsessions and compulsions. *Biological Psychiatry*, **20**, 1117.

Curran J.P. (1973) Tardive dyskinesia: side-effect or not? *American Journal of Psychiatry*, **130**, 406–10.

Curry S.H. (1971) Chlorpromazine: concentration in plasma, excretion in urine and duration of effect. *Proceedings of the Royal Society of Medicine*, **64**, 285–9.

Curson D.A., Pantelis C., Ward J. & Barnes T.R.E. (1992) Institutionalism and schizophrenia 30 years on. Clinical poverty and the social environment in three British mental hospitals in 1960 compared with a fourth in 1990. *British Journal of Psychiatry*, **160**, 230–41.

Cutler N.R., Post R.M., Rey A.C. & Bunney W.E. (1981) Depression-dependent dyskinesias in two cases of manic–depressive illness. *New England Journal of Medicine*, **304**, 1088–9.

Damasio D.R., Damasio H. & Chui H.C. (1980) Neglect following damage to frontal lobe or basal ganglia. *Neuropsychologia*, **18**, 123–32.

De U.J. (1973) Catatonia from fluphenazine. *British Journal of Psychiatry*, **122**, 240–1.

Degkwitz R. (1969) Extrapyramidal motor disorders following long-term treatment with neuroleptic drugs. In: G.E. Crane & R. Gardner (Eds.), *Psychotropic Drugs and Dysfunctions of the Basal Ganglia*. Washington: US Public Health Service Publication No. 1938, pp. 22–5.

Delay J. & Deniker P. (1956) Chlorpromazine and neuroleptic treatments in psychiatry. *Journal of Clinical and Experimental Psychopathology and Quarterly Review of Psychiatry and Neurology*, **17**, 19–24.

Delay J. & Deniker P. (1960) Apport de la clinique a la connaissance de l'action des neuroleptiques. *Revue Canadienne de Biologie*, **20**, 397–423.

Delbeke R. & Bogaert L van (1928) Le probleme general des crises oculogyres au cours de l'encephalite epidemique chronique. *L'encephale*, **23**, 855–90.

Denckla M.B. (1989) Neurological Examination. In: J.L. Rapoport (Ed.), *Obsessive Compulsive Disorder in Children and Adolescents*, pp. 107–19. America Psychiatric Press Inc.: Washington.

Denham J. & Carrick D.J.E.L. (1959–60) Therapeutic importance of extrapyramidal phenomena evoked by a new phenothiazine. *American Journal of Psychiatry*, **116**, 927–8.

Deniker P. (1960) Experimental neurological syndromes and the new drug therapies in psychiatry. *Comprehensive Psychiatry*, **1**, 92–102.

Denny-Brown D. (1950) Disintegration of motor function resulting from cerebral lesions. *Journal of Nervous and Mental Disease*, **112**, 1–45.

Denny-Brown D. (1958) The nature of apraxia. *Journal of Nervous and Mental Disease*, **126**, 9–32.

Denny-Brown D (1968) Clinical symptomatology of diseases of the basal ganglia. In: P.J. Vinken & G.W. Bruyn (Eds.), *Handbook of Clinical Neurology, Vol. 6 Diseases of the Basal Ganglia* North-Holland Publishing Co: Amsterdam.

Dide, Guiraud & Lafage (1921) Syndrome parkinsonien dans la demence precoce. *Revue Neurologique*, **28**, 692–4.

Divry P. (1928) La catatonie. *Session du Congres des Medecins Alienistes et Neurologistes, Anvers*. Quoted in Vermeylen (1938).

Dretler J. (1935) Influence de l'encephalite epidemique sur la schizophrenie. *Encephale*, **30**, 656–70.

Earl C.J. (1934) The primitive catatonic psychosis of idiocy. *British Journal of Medical Psychology*, **14**, 111–230.

Earl C.J. (1983) Personal communication.

Economo C. von (1931) *Encephalitis Lethargica, its Sequelae and Treatment*, translated by K.O. Newman. Oxford University Press: London.

Elliot T.R. (1904) On the action of adrenalin. *Journal of Physiology*, **31**, 20–2.

Fahn S. (1983)   Treatment of tardive dyskinesia, use of dopamine depleting drugs. *Clinical Neuropharmacology*, **6**, 151–8.

Fahn S., Williams D., Lesser R.P., Jankovic J. & Silberstein S.D. (1983)   Hysterical dystonia, a rare disorder: report of five documented cases. *Neurology*, **33** (suppl 2), 161.

Fallon J.R. & Moore R.Y. (1978)   Catecholamine innervation of the basal forebrain IV. Topography of the dopamine projection to the basal forebrain and neostriatum. *Journal of Comp. Neurology*, **180**, 545–80.

Farran-Ridge C. (1926)   Some symptoms referable to the basal ganglia occurring in dementia praecox and epidemic encephalitis. *Journal of Mental Science*, **72**, 513–23.

Fish F. (1964)   The influence of the tranquillisers on the Leonhard schizophrenic syndromes. *Encephale*, **1**, 245–9.

Fishbain D.A., Goldberg M., Khalil T.M., Asfour S.S., Abdel-Moty E., Meagher B.R., Santana R., Rosomoff R.S. & Rosomoff H.L. (1988)   The utility of electromyographic biofeedback in the treatment of conversion paralysis. *American Journal of Psychiatry*, **145**, 1572–5.

Fisher C.M. (1983)   Abulia minor vs. agitated behaviour. *Clinical Neurosurgery*, **31**, 9–31.

Forbes T.W. (1934)   Studies of catatonia. II. Central control of cerea flexibilitas. III. Bodily postures assumed while sleeping. *The Psychiatric Quarterly*, **8**, 538–45, 546–52.

Ford R.A. (1989)   The psychopathology of echophenomena. *Psychological Medicine*, **19**, 627–35.

Freeman T. & Gathercole C.E. (1966)   Perseveration—the clinical symptoms—in chronic schizophrenia and organic dementia. *British Journal of Psychiatry*, **112**, 27–32.

Freyhan F.A. (1957)   Psychomotility and parkinsonism in treatment with neuroleptic drugs. *Archives of Neurology and Psychiatry*, **78**, 465–72.

Fricchione G.L. (1985)   Neuroleptic catatonia and its relationship to psychogenic catatonia. *Biological Psychiatry*, **20**, 304–13.

Friedman A.S. (1964)   Minimal effects of severe depression on cognitive functioning. *Journal of Abnormal and Social Psychology*, **69**, 237–43.

Frith C.D. & Done D.J. (1986)   Stereotyped behaviour in madness and in health. In: S.J. Cooper & C.T. Dourish (Eds.), *The Neurobiology of Behavioural Stereotypy*. Oxford University Press: Oxford.

Gelenberg A.J. (1976)   The catatonic syndrome. *Lancet*, i, 1339–41.

Gelenberg A.J. & Mandel M.R. (1977)   Catatonic reactions to high-potency neuroleptic drugs. *Archives of General Psychiatry*, **34**, 947–50.

Gietke H., Thier P. & Bolz J. (1981)   The relationship between P3-latency and reaction time in depression. *Biological Psychology*, **13**, 31–49.

Girgis M. & Kiloh L.G. (Eds.) (1980)   *Limbic Epilepsy and the Dyscontrol Syndrome*. Elsevier/North Holland Biomedical Press: Amsterdam.

Gjessing R.R. (1976) *Contribution to the Somatology of Periodic Catatonia.* Pergamon Press: Oxford.

Glazer W.M., Morgenstern H., Schooler N., Berkman C.S. & Moore D.C. (1990) Predictors of improvement in tardive dyskinesia following discontinuation of neuroleptic medication. *British Journal of Psychiatry*, **157**, 585–92.

Godfrey H.P.D. & Knight R.G. (1984) The validity of actometer and speech activity measures in the assessment of depressed patients. *British Journal of Psychiatry*, **145**, 159–63.

Goode D.J., Manning A.A., Middleton J.F. & Williams B. (1981) Fine motor performance before and after treatment in schizophrenia and schizo-affective patients. *Psychiatry Research*, **5**, 247–55.

Goodwin F.K., Brodie H.K.H., Murphy D.L. & Bunney W.E. (1970) Administration of a peripheral decarboxylase inhibitor with L-dopa to depressed patients. *Lancet*, **i**, 908–11.

Gould R., Miller B.L., Goldberg M.A. & Benson D.F. (1986) The validity of hysterical signs and symptoms. *The Journal of Nervous and Mental Disease*, **174**, 593–7.

Greden J.F. & Carroll B.J. (1981) Psychomotor function in active disorders: an overview of new monitoring techniques. *American Journal of Psychiatry*, **138**, 1441–8.

Greden J.F., Albala A.A., Smokler I.A., Gardner R. & Carroll B.J. (1981) Speech pause time: a marker of psychomotor retardation among endogenous depressives. *Biological Psychiatry*, **16**, 851–9.

Griesinger W. (1845) *Die Pathologie und Therapie der psychischen Krankheiten.* Krabbe: Stuttgart.

Guenther W., Guenther R., Streck P., Romig H. & Rodel A. (1988) Psychomotor disturbances in psychiatric patients as a possible basis for new attempts at differential diagnosis and therapy. III. Cross validation study on depressed patients: the psychotic motor syndrome as a possible state marker for endogenous depression. *European Archives of Psychiatry and Neurological Sciences*, **237**, 65–73.

Guggenheim F.G. & Babigian H.M. (1974) Catatonic schizophrenia: epidemiology and clinical course. *Journal of Nervous and Mental Diseases*, **158**, 291–305.

Guiraud P. (1924) Conception neurologique du syndrome catatonique. *Encephale*, **19**, 571–9.

Guiraud P. (1936) Analyse duo symptome stereotype. *Encephale*, **31**, 229–70.

Guy W. (1976) Abnormal involuntary movement scale. *ECDEU Assessment Manual for Psychopharmacology.* U.S. Department of Health, Education and Welfare, Public Health Service, Alcohol, Drug abuse, and Mental Health administration: Rockville, MD 20852.

Haase H.-J. (1958) La valeur therapeutique des symptomes extrapyramidaux dans le traitement a la chlorpromazine et reserpine. *Encephale*, **48**, 519–32.

Haase H.-J. (1961)   Extrapyramidal modifications of fine movements—a 'conditio sine qua non' of the fundamental therapeutic action neuroleptic drugs. *Revue Canadienne de Biologie*, **20**, 425–49.

Hall K.R.L. & Stride E. (1952)   Some factors affecting reaction times to auditory stimuli in mental patients. *Journal of Mental Science*, **100**, 462–77.

Hamilton M. (1960)   A rating scale for depression. *Journal of Neurology, Neurosurgery and Psychiatry*, **23**, 56–62.

Hardy P., Jouvent R. & Widlocher D. (1984)   Speech pause time and the retardation rating scale for depression (ERD); towards a reciprocal validation. *Journal of Affective Disorders*, **6**, 123–7.

Hart B. (1932)   Psychology and psychiatry. *Proceedings of the Royal Society of Medicine*, **25**, 187–200.

Haskovec L. (1901)   L'akathisie. *Revue Neurologique*, **9**, 1107–9.

Haskovec L. (1925)   Le psychisme sous-cortical. *Revue Neurologique*, **1**, 976–88.

Helms P.M. & Godwin C.D. (1985)   Abnormalities of blink rate in psychoses: a preliminary report. *Biological Psychiatry*, **20**, 94–119.

Hicks L.H. & Birren J.E. (1970)   Aging, brain damage, and psychomotor slowing. *Psychological Bulletin*, **74**, 377–96.

Hoffman A.S. (1986)   Catatonic reaction to accidental haloperidol overdose: an unrecognised drug abuse risk. *Journal of Nervous and Mental Disease*, **174**, 428–30.

Hoffmann G.M.A., Gonze J.C. & Mendlewicz J. (1985)   Speech pause time as a method for the evaluation of psychomotor retardation in depressive illness. *British Journal of Psychiatry*, **146**, 535–8.

Hogarty G.E. & Gross M. (1966)   Preadmission symptom differences between first-admitted schizophrenics in the predrug and postdrug era. *Comprehensive Psychiatry*, **7**, 134–40.

Hollander E., Schiffman E., Cohen B., Rivera-Stein M.A., Rosen W., Gorman J.M., Fyer A.J., Papp L. & Liebowitz M.R. (1990)   Signs of central nervous system dysfunction in obsessive–compulsive disorder. *Archives of General Psychiatry*, **47**, 27–32.

Holzman P.S., Proctor L.R. & Hughes D.W. (1973)   Eye tracking patterns in schizophrenia. *Science*, **181**, 179–81.

Hunter R., Earl C.J. & Thornicroft S. (1964)   An apparently irreversible syndrome of abnormal movements following phenothiazine medication. *Proceedings of the Royal Society of Medicine*, **57**, 758–62.

Hunter R. & Macalpine I. (1974)   *Psychiatry for the Poor*. Dawsons: Pall Mall.

Hymas N. & Prasad A.J. (1989)   Obsessive–compulsive disorder: its clinical neurology and recent pharmacological studies. In: A.J. Prasad (Ed.), *Biological Basis and Therapy of Neuroses*, pp. 41–79. CRC Press Inc: Boca Raton.

Hymas N., Lees A., Bolton D., Epps K. & Head D. (1991)   The neurology of obsessional slowness. *Brain*, **114**, 2203–33.

Iacono W.G., Tuason V.B. & Johnson R.A. (1981)   Dissociation of smooth-pursuit and saccadic eye tracking in remitted schizophrenics. *Archives of General Psychiatry*, **38**, 991–6.

Janet P. (1903) *Les Obsessions et la Psychasthenie*. Alcan: Paris.

Jankovic J. & Orman J. (1987) Botulinum a toxin for cranial–cervical dystonia: a double-blind placebo controlled study. *Neurology*, **37**, 616–23.

Javoy-Agid F. & Agid Y. (1980) Is the mesocortical dopaminergic system involved in Parkinson's disease? *Neurology*, **30**, 1326–31.

Jawed S.H. & Singh I. (1989) Tardive dyskinesia with schizophrenic relapse. *Journal of Mental Deficiency Research*, **33**, 331–4.

Jayne D., Lees A.J. & Stern G.M. (1984) Remission in spasmodic torticollis. *Journal of Neurology, Neurosurgery and Psychiatry*, **47**, 1236–7.

Jelliffe S.E. (1927) The mental pictures in schizophrenia and in epidemic encephalitis, their alliances, differences and a point of view. *American Journal of Psychiatry*, **6**, 413–65.

Jelliffe S.E. (1929) Oculogyric crises as compulsion phenomena in postencephalitis: their occurrence, phenomenology and meaning. *Journal of Nervous and Mental Diseases*, **69**, 59–68, 165–84, 278–97, 415–26, 531–51 and 666–79.

Jelliffe S.E. (1932) *Psychopathology of Forced Movements and the Oculogyric Crises of Lethargic Encephalitis*. Nervous & Mental Disease Publishing Co: Washington.

Jelliffe S.E. (1940) The parkinsonian body posture, some considerations of unconscious hostility. *Psychoanalytic Review*, **27**, 467–79.

Jelliffe S.E. & White W.A. (1917) *Diseases of the Nervous System. A Text-book of Neurology and Psychiatry*. Lea & Febiger: Philadelphia.

Jeste D.V. & Wyatt R.J. (1982) Therapeutic strategies against tardive dyskinesia, two decades of experience. *Archives of General Psychiatry*, **39**, 803–16.

Johnson J. & Lucey P.A. (1987) Encephalitis lethargica, a contemporary cause of catatonic stupor. A report of two cases. *British Journal of Psychiatry*, **151**, 550–2.

Johnstone E.C., Owens D.G.C., Gold A., Crow T.J. & Macmillan J.F. (1981) Institutionalization and the defects of schizophrenia. *British Journal of Psychiatry*, **139**, 195–203.

Jones I.H. (1965) Observations on schizophrenic stereotypies. *Comprehensive Psychiatry*, **6**, 323–35.

Jones M. & Hunter R. (1969) Abnormal movements in patients with chronic psychiatric illness. In: G.E. Crane & J. Gardner (Eds.), *Psychotropic Drugs and Dysfunctions of the Basal Ganglia*. NIMH, Bethesda, Public Health Service publication no. 1938.

Jouvent R., Frechette D., Binoux F., Lancrenon S. & des Lauriers A. (1980) Le ralentissement psycho-moteur dans les etats depressifs: construction d'une echelle d'evaluation quantitative. *Encephale*, **VI**, 41–58.

Joyston-Bechal M.P. (1966) The clinical features and outcome of stupor. *British Journal of Psychiatry*, **112**, 967–81.

Kahlbaum K. (1874) *Die Katatonie oder das Spannungs-Irresein*. Hirschwald: Berlin. (1973) *Catatonia*, translated by Y. Levij & T. Priden, John Hopkins University Press: Baltimore.

Kahn E. and Cohen L.H. (1934)   Organic drivenness: a brain-stem syndrome and an experience. *New England Journal of Medicine*, **210**, 748–56.

Kalachnik J.E. (1984)   Tardive dyskinesia and the mentally retarded: a review. In S.E. Breuning (Ed.), *Advances in Mental Retardation and Developmental Disabilities*, Vol. 2, pp. 329–56. JAI Press: London.

Kanzler N. & Malitz S. (1972)   L-dopa for the treatment of depression. In: S. Malitz (Ed.), *L-dopa and Behaviour*, pp. 103–19. Raven Press: New York.

Karson C.N. (1979)   Oculomotor signs in a psychiatric population: a preliminary report. *American Journal of Psychiatry*, **136**, 1057–60.

Karson C.N. (1983)   Spontaneous eye-blink rates and dopaminergic systems. *Brain*, **106**, 643–53.

Karson C.N., Bigelow, L.B., Kleinman J.E., Weinberger D. & Wyatt R.J. (1982)   Haloperidol-induced changes in blink rates correlate with changes in BPRS score. *British Journal of Psychiatry*, **140**, 503–7.

Karson C.N., Dykman R.A. & Paige S.R. (1990)   Blink rates in schizophrenia. *Schizophrenia Bulletin*, **16**, 345–54.

Keane J.R. (1986)   Wrong-way deviation of the tongue with hysterical hemiparesis. *Neurology*, **36**, 1406–7.

Keane J.R. (1989)   Hysterical gait disorders: 60 cases. *Neurology*, **39**, 586–9.

Kellam A.M.P. (1990)   The (frequently) neuroleptic (potentially) malignant syndrome. *British Journal of Psychiatry*, **157**, 169–73.

Keshavan M.S. & Goswamy W. (1983)   Tardive dyskinesia less severe in depression. *British Journal of Psychiatry*, **142**, 207–8.

Kiloh L.G. (1961)   Pseudo-dementia. *Acta Psychiatrical Scandinavica*, **37**, 336–51.

King H.E. (1954)   *Psychomotor Aspects of Motor Disease. An Experimental Study*. Harvard University Press: Cambridge Mass.

Kirby G.H. (1913)   The catatonic syndrome and its relation to manic-depressive insanity. *Journal of Nervous and Mental Diseases*, **40**, 694–704.

Klawans H.L. (1983)   Introduction, symposium on tardive dyskinesia. *Clinical Neuropharmacology*, **6**, 75.

Klawans H.L., Goetz C. & Westheimer R. (1972)   Pathophysiology of schizophrenia and the striatum. *Diseases of the Nervous System*, **33**, 711–9.

Klawans H.L., Bergen B., Bruyn G.W. & Paulson G.W. (1974)   Neuroleptic-induced tardive dyskinesias in nonpsychotic patients. *Archives of Neurology*, **30**, 338–9.

Klee A. (1961)   Akinetic mutism: review of the literature and report of a case. *Journal of Nervous and Mental Disease*, **133**, 536–53.

Kleinman J.E., Karson C.N., Weinberger D.R., Freed W.J., Berman K.F. & Wyatt R.J. (1984)   Eye-blinking and cerebral ventricular size in chronic schizophrenic patients. *American Journal of Psychiatry*, **141**, 1430–2.

Kleist K. (1960)   Schizophrenic symptoms and cerebral pathology. *Journal of Mental Science*, **106**, 246–55.

Kline N. & Mettler F. (1961)   The extrapyramidal system and schizophrenia. *Revue Canadienne de Biologie*, **20**, 583–7.

Knott V.J. & Lapierre Y.D. (1987)   Electrophysiological and behavioral correlates of psychomotor responsivity in depression. *Biological Psychiatry*, **22**, 313–24.

Koller W., Lang A., Vetere-Overfield B., Findley L, Cleeves L., Factor S., Singer C. & Weiner W. (1989)   Psychogenic tremors. *Neurology*, **39**, 1094–9.

Koshino Y., Wada Y., Isaki K. & Kurata K. (1991)   A long-term outcome study of tardive dyskinesia in patients on antipsychotic medication. *Clinical Neuropharmacology*, **14**, 537–46.

Kraepelin E. (1919) *Dementia Praecox and Paraphrenia*, translated by R. Barclay. Livingstone: Edinburgh.

Kruse W. (1957)   Parkinsonism, schizophrenia and ataractic drugs. *Diseases of the Nervous System*, **18**, 474–7.

Kuhn T.S. (1970) *The Structure of Scientific Revolutions*, 2nd edn. University of Chicago Press: Chicago.

Kupfer D.J., Weiss B.L., Foster F.G., Detre T.P., Delgado J. & McPartland R. (1974)   Psychomotor activity in affective states. *Archives of General Psychiatry*, **30**, 765–8.

Kyriakides T. & Hewer R.L. (1988)   Hand contractures in Parkinson's disease. *Journal of Neurology, Neurosurgery and Psychiatry*, **51**, 1221–3.

Lal K.P., Saxena S. & Mohan D. (1988)   Tardive dystonia alternating with mania. *Biological Psychiatry*, **23**, 312–6.

Lange J. (1922) Katatonische Erscheinungen im Rahmen manischer Erkrankungen. In: Alzheimer A., Lewandowsky (Eds.), *Monographien aus dem Gestamtgebiete der Neurologie und Psychiatrie*, no. 31. Julius Springer: Berlin.

Laplane D. & Degos J.D. (1983)   Motor neglect. *Journal of Neurology, Neurosurgery, and Psychiatry*, **46**, 152–8.

Laplane D., Baulac M., Widlocher D. & Dubois B. (1984)   Pure psychic akinesia with bilateral lesions of basal ganglia. *Journal of Neurology, Neurosurgery, and Psychiatry*, **47**, 377–85.

Laplane D., Levasseur M., Pillon B., Dubois B., Baulac M., Mazoyer B., Dinh S.T., Sette G., Danze F. & Baron J.C. (1989)   Obsessive-compulsive and other behavioural changes with bilateral basal ganglia lesions. *Brain*, **112**, 699–725.

Lewis A. (1934a)   Melancholia: a historical review. *Journal of Mental Science*, **80**, 1–42.

Lewis A. (1934b)   Melancholia: a clinical survey of depressive states. *Journal of Mental Science*, **80**, 278–378.

Lewis A. & Minski L. (1935)   Chorea and psychosis. *Lancet*, i, 536–8.

Lewy F.H. (1942)   Historical Introduction. In: Putnam T.J., Frantz A.M. & Ranson S.W. (Eds.) *The Diseases of the Basal Ganglia*, pp. 1–20. Williams & Wilkins: Baltimore.

Lhermitte F. (1983)   'Utilisation behaviour' and its relation to lesions of the frontal lobes. *Brain*, **106**, 237–55.

Lilly R., Cummings J.L., Benson D.F. & Frankel M. (1983)   The human Kluver–Bucy syndrome. *Neurology*, **33**, 1141–5.

Ljungeberg L. (1957)   Hysteria. A clinical, prognostic and genetic study. *Acta Psychiatrica et Neurologica Scandinavica*, **32**(suppl. 112), 1–162.

Luchins D.J. (1990)   A possible role of hippocampal dysfunction in schizophrenic symptomatology. *Biological Psychiatry*, **28**, 87–91.

Lund C.E., Mortimer A.M., Rogers D. and McKenna P.J. (1991)   Motor, volitional and behavioural disorders in schizophrenia 1: Assessment using the modified Rogers scale. *British Journal of Psychiatry*, **158**, 323–7.

Mackert A., Woyth C., Flechtner K.-M. & Volt H.-P. (1990)   Increased blink rate psychiatric illness. *Biological Psychiatry*, **27**, 1197–202.

Mackintosh J.H., Kumar R. & Kitamura T. (1983)   Blink rate in psychiatric illness. *British Journal of Psychiatry*, **143**, 55–7.

Magoun H.W. (1950)   Caudal and cephalic influences of the brain-stem reticular formation. *Physiological Review*, **30**, 459–74.

Mahendra B. (1981)   Where have all the catatonics gone? *Psychological Medicine*, **11**, 669–71.

Manschreck T.C. (1983)   Psychopathology of motor behavior in schizophrenia. *Progress in Experimental Personality Research*, **12**, 53–99.

Manschreck T.C., Maher B.A., Rucklos M.E. & Vereen D.R. (1982)   Disturbed voluntary motor activity in schizophrenic disorder. *Psychological Medicine*, **12**, 73–84.

Manschreck T.C., Maher B.A., Waller N.G., Ames D. & Latham C.A. (1985)   Deficient motor synchrony in schizophrenic disorders: clinical correlates. *Biological Psychiatry*, **20**, 990–1002.

Manschreck T.C., Keuthen N.J. Schneyer N.L., Celada M.T., Laughery J. & Collins P. (1990)   Abnormal involuntary movements and chronic schizophrenic disorders. *Biological Psychiatry*, **27**, 150–8.

Marinesco G. & Radovici A. (1926)   Des rapports de l'encephalite epidemique avec certains troubles hysteriques. *Journal de Neurologie et Psychiatrie*, **26**, 259–68.

Markham C.H. (1973)   Essay on akinesia. In: J. Siegfried (Ed.), *Parkinson's Disease. Rigidity—Akinesia—Behavior* pp. 207–12. Hans Huber: Bern.

Marsden C.D. (1976)   Dystonia: the spectrum of the disease. In: M.D. Yahr (Ed.), *The Basal Ganglia*, pp. 351–67. Raven Press: New York.

Marsden C.D. (1982)   Motor disorders in schizophrenia. *Psychological Medicine*, **12**, 13–5.

Marsden C.D. (1986)   Hysteria—a neurologist's view. *Psychological Medicine*, **16**, 277–88.

Marsden C.D., Tarsy D. & Baldesserini R.J. (1975)   Spontaneous and drug-induced movement disorders in psychotic patients. In: D.F. Benson & D. Blumer (Eds.), *Psychiatric Aspects of Neurological Disease*, pp. 219–65. Grune & Stratton: New York.

Martin I. & Rees I. (1966)   Reaction times and somatic reactivity in depressed patients. *Journal of Psychosomatic Research*, **9**, 375–82.

Martin J.P. (1983)   Old photographs: postencephalitic Parkinsonism in two small boys. *Journal of Neurology, Neurosurgery and Psychiatry*, **46**, 953–5.

Martin J.P., Hurwitz L.J. & Finlayson M.H. (1962)   The negative symptom of basal gangliar disease. *Lancet*, **ii**, 1–6, 62–6.

Matussek N., Benkert O., Schneider K., Otten H. & Pohlmeier H. (1970) L-dopa plus decarboxylase inhibitor in depression. *Lancet*, **ii**, 660–1.

Maudsley H. (1873)   *Body and Mind: an Enquiry into their Connection and Mutual Influence, Specially in Reference to Mental Disorders*. Macmillan: London.

May R.H. (1959)   Catatonic-like states following phenothiazine therapy. *American Journal of Psychiatry*, **115**, 1119–20.

McCarthy J.A. (1979)   Unusual phenomenon in Parkinson's disease. *Annals of Neurology*, **5**, 499.

McClelland H.A., Metcalfe A.V., Kerr T.A., Dutta D. & Watson P. (1991) Facial dyskinesia: a 16-year follow-up study. *British Journal of Psychiatry*, **158**, 691–6.

McCreadie R.G., Barron E.T. & Winslow G.S. (1982)   The Nithsdale schizophrenia survey: II. Abnormal movements. *British Journal of Psychiatry*, **140**, 587–90.

McCurdy J. T. (1925)   *The Psychology of Emotion*. Kegan Paul: London.

McKenna P.J., Lund C.E., Mortimer C.E. & Biggins C.A. (1991)   Motor, volitional and behavioural disorders in schizophrenia. 2: The 'conflict of paradigms' hypothesis. *British Journal of Psychiatry*, **158**, 328–36.

Meier-Koll & Pohl P. (1979)   Chronobiological aspects of stereotyped motor behaviour in mentally retarded children. *International Journal of Chronobiology*, **6**, 191–209.

Meige H. (1905)   *Tics*. Monographies Cliniques, Masson: Paris.

Meiselas K.D., Spencer E.K., Oberfield R., Peselow E., Angrist B. & Campbell M. (1989)   Differentiation of stereotypies from neuroleptic-related dyskinesias in autistic children. *Journal of Clinical Psychopharmacology*, **9**, 207–9.

Mettler F. (1955)   Perceptual capacity, functioning of the corpus striatum and schizophrenia. *Psychiatric Quarterly*, **29**, 89–111.

Miller E. (1927)   Metnal dissociation: its relation to catatonia and the mechanism of narcolepsy. *Brain*, **50**, 624–30.

Mori E. & Yamadori A. (1989)   Rejection behaviour: a human homologue of the abnormal behaviour of Denny-Brown and Chambers' monkey with bilateral parietal ablation. *Journal of Neurology, Neurosurgery and Psychiatry*, **52**, 1260–66.

Morrison J.R. (1973)   Catatonia: retarded and excited types. *Archives of General Psychiatry*, **28**, 39–41.

Morrison J.R. (1974)   Changes in subtype diagnosis of schizophrenia: 1920–1966. *American Journal of Psychiatry*, **131**, 674–7.

Nadel C. (1978)   Tardive dyskinesia or schizophrenic abnormal movements. *British Journal of Psychiatry*, **133**, 287–8.

Naville F. (1922)   Etudes sur les complications et les sequelles mentales de l'encephalite epidemique: la bradyphrenie. *Encephale*, **17**, 369–75, 423–36.

Nelson J.C. & Charney D.S. (1981)   The symptoms of major depressive illness. *American Journal of Psychiatry*, **138**, 1.

Nielson J.M. (1936)   Extreme encephalitic parkinsonism with contractures which relax during somnambulstic state. *Bulletin of Los Angeles Neurological Society*, **1**, 28–30.

Nilsonne A. (1988)   Speech characteristics as indicators of depressive illness. Acta Psychiatrica Scandinavica, **77**, 253–63.

Norman H.J. (1928)   *Mental Disorders, a Handbook for Students and Practitioners*. Livingstone: Edinburgh.

O'Gorman G. (1979)   Abnormalities of movement. In: James F.E. & Snaith R.P. (Eds.), *Psychiatric Illness and Mental Handicap*, pp. 91–101. Gaskell Press: London.

Ojemann G.A. (1982)   Interrelationships in the localisation of language, memory, and motor mechanisms in human cortex and thalamus. In: R.A. Thomson and J.R. Green (Eds.), *New Perspectives in Cerebral Localisation*, pp. 157–75. Raven Press: New York.

Orton (1930)   Some neurologic concepts applied to schizophrenia. *Archives of Neurology and Psychiatry*, **23**, 114–29.

Ostow M. & Ostow M. (1946)   The frequency of blinking in mental illness: a measurable somatic aspect of attitude. *Journal of Nervous and Mental Disease*, **102**, 294–301.

Owens D.G.C., Johnstone E.C. & Frith C.D. (1982)   Spontaneous involuntary disorders of movement: their prevalence, severity, and distribution in chronic schizophrenics with and without treatment with neuroleptics. *Archives of General Psychiatry*, **39**, 452–61.

Pauls D.L., Towbin K.E., Leckman J.F., Zahner G.E.P. & Cohen D.J. (1986)   Gilles de la Tourette syndrome and obsessive–compulsive disorder: evidence supporting a genetic relationship. *Archives of General Psychiatry*, **43**, 1180–2.

Payne R.W. & Hewlett J.H.G. (1960)   Thought disorder in psychotic patients. In: H.J. Eysenck (Ed.), *Experiments in Personality*, Vol. II, pp. 3–104. Routledge & Kegan Paul: London.

Penfield W. (1958)   *The Excitable Cortex in Conscious Man*. Liverpool University Press: Liverpool.

Perez-Sales P. (1990)   Camptocormia. *British Journal of Psychiatry*, **157**, 765–7.

Pienkowsi S.K. (1925)   La valeur des etudes de Charcot sur les troubles moteurs de l'hysterie au point de vue de la pathophysiologie de la motilite. *Revue Neurologique*, **1**, 988–93.

Pitman R., Green R.C., Jenike M.A. & Mesulam M.M. (1987)   Clinical comparison of Tourette syndrome and obsessive–compulsive disorder. *American Journal of Psychiatry*, **144**, 1161–71.

Power R.W., Linkowski P. & Mendlewicz J. (1983)   State-dependent tardive dyskinesia in manic-depressive illness. *Journal of Neurology, Neurosurgery and Psychiatry*, **46**, 666–8.

Price K.S., Farley I.J. & Horneykiewicz O. (1978) Neurochemistry of Parkinson's disease: relation between striatal and limbic dopamine. In: P.J. Roberts, G.N. Woodruff & L.L. Iverson (Eds.), *Dopamine: Advances in Biochemical Psychopharmacology*, Vol. 19, pp. 293–300. Raven Press: New York.

Proceedings of the First International Congress of Neuropathology, Vol. 3, (1952) Rosenberg & Sellier: Turin.

Rachman S. (1974) Primary obsessional slowness. *Behaviour Research and Therapy*, **12**, 9–18.

Radovici M.A. (1930) L'hysterie et les etats hysteroides organiques. *Revue Neurologique*, **1**, 1163–74.

Reiter P.J. (1926) Extrapyramidal disturbances in dementia praecox. *Acta Psychiatrica et Neurologica*, **1**, 287–305.

Richardson M.A., Haugland G., Pass R. & Craig T.J. (1986) The prevalence of tardive dyskinesia in a mentally retarded population. *Psychopharmacology Bulletin*, **22**, 243–9.

Ridley R.M. & Baker H.F. (1982) Stereotypy in monkeys and humans. *Psychological Medicine*, **12**, 61–72.

Ries R.K. (1985) DSMIII implications of the diagnoses of catatonia and bipolar disorder. *American Journal of Psychiatry*, **142**, 1471–4.

Robinson A.D.T. & McCreadie R.G. (1986) The Nithsdale schizophrenia survey V. Follow-up of tardive dyskinesia at $3\frac{1}{2}$ years. *British Journal of Psychiatry*, **149**, 621–3.

Robinson B.W. (1976) Limbic influences on human speech. *Annals of the New York Academy of Science*, **280**, 761–71.

Rogers D. (1985) The motor disorders of severe psychiatric illness: a conflict of paradigms. *British Journal of Psychiatry*, **147**, 221–32.

Rogers D. (1986) Bradyphrenia in parkinsonism: a historical review. *Psychological Medicine*, **16**, 257–65.

Rogers D. (1988) Psychiatry and the Necker cube. Neurological and psychological conceptions of psychiatric disorder. *Behavioural Neurology*, Vol. 1. Clinical Neurosciences Publications: Oxford, pp. 3–10.

Rogers D. (1989a) Neurosis and neurological disorder. In: A.J. Prasad (Ed.), *Biological Basis and Therapy of Neuroses*, pp. 145–58. CRC Press Inc: Boca Raton.

Rogers D. (1989b) Oculogyric crises and schizophrenia. *British Journal of Psychiatry*, **155**, 569–70.

Rogers D. (1990) Psychiatric consequences of basal ganglia disease. *Seminars in Neurology*, **10**, 262–6.

Rogers D. (1991) Catatonia: a contemporary approach. *Journal of Neuropsychiatry*, **3**, 334–40.

Rogers D., Lees A.J., Smith E., Trimble M. & Stern G.M. (1987) Bradyphrenia in Parkinson's disease and psychomotor retardation in depressive illness: an experimental study. *Brain*, **110**, 761–76.

Rogers D., Karki C., Bartlett C. & Pocock P. (1991) The motor disorder of mental handicap: an overlap with the motor disorders of severe psychiatric illness. *British Journal of Psychiatry*, **158**, 97–102.

Rolak L.A. (1988) Psychogenic sensory loss. *The Journal of Nervous and Mental Disease*, **176**, 686–7.

Ron M.A. & Harvey I. (1990) Editorial: the brain in schizophrenia. *Journal of Neurology, Neurosurgery and Psychiatry*, **53**, 725–6.

Rosner A.A. (1942) Unit reaction states in oculogyric crises. *American Journal of Psychiatry*, **99**, 224–8.

Royant-Parola S., Borbely A.A., Tobler I., Benoit O. & Widlocher D. (1986) Monitoring of long-term motor activity in depressed patients. *British Journal of Psychiatry*, **149**, 288–93.

Sachdev P.S. (1989) Depression-dependent exacerbation of tardive dyskinesia. *British Journal of Psychiatry*, **155**, 253–5.

Salmon A. (1950) Le cerveau organique comme le siege principal des phenomemenes hysteriques. *Encephale*, **39**, 511–22.

Sawle G.V., Hymas N.F., Lees A.J. & Frackowiak R.S.J. (1991) Obsessional slowness: functional studies with positron emission tomography. *Brain*, **114**, 2191–202.

Schilder P. (1938) The organic background of obsessions and compulsions. *American Journal of Psychiatry*, **94**, 1397–416.

Schlegel S., Maier W., Phillipp M., Heuser I. & Aldenoff J. (1988) The association between psychopathological aspects and CT measurements in affective disorders. *Pharmacopsychiatry (Stuttgart)*, **21**, 416–7.

Schneider J.S. (1984) Basal ganglia role in behaviour: importance of sensory gating and its importance to psychiatry. *Biological Psychiatry*, **19**, 1693–710.

Schonecker M. (1957) A strange syndrome in the oral area with application of chlorpromazine. *Nervenarzt*, **28**, 35.

Schwab R.S. & Zieper I. (1965) Effects of mood, motivation, stress and alertness on the performance in Parkinson's disease. *Psychiatria et Neurologia (Basel)*, **150**, 345–57.

Shakow D. & Huston P.E. (1936) Studies of motor function in schizophrenia: 1. Speed of tapping. *Journal of General Psychology*, **15**, 63–103.

Shapiro M.B. & Nelson E.H. (1955) An investigation of the nature of cognitive impairment in co-operative psychiatric patients. *British Journal of Medical Psychology*, **28**, 239–56.

Sigwald J., Bouttier D. & Courvoisier S. (1959a) Les accidents neurologiques des medications neuroleptiques. *Revue Neurologique*, **100**, 553–95.

Sigwald J., Bouttier D., Raymondeau C. & Piot C. (1959b) Quatre cas de dyskinesie facio-bucco-linguo-masticatrice a evolution prolongee secondaire a un traitement par les neuroleptiques. *Revue Neurologique*, **100**, 751–5.

Simpson G.M. & Kunz-Bartholini E. (1968) Relationship of individual tolerance, behavior and phenothiazine produced extrapyramidal system disturbance. *Diseases of the Nervous System*, **29**, 269–74.

Simpson G.M. & Angus J.W.S. (1970) Drug-induced extrapyramidal disorders. *Acta Psychiatrica Scandinavica*, supplementum **212**, 1–58.

Simpson G.M., Lee J.H., Zoubok B. & Gardos G.L. (1979) A rating scale for tardive dyskinesia. *Psychopharmacology*, **64**, 171–9.

Slater E. (1965) Diagnosis of 'hysteria'. *British Medical Journal*, **1**, 1395–9.

Smith S. (1959) An investigation and survey of akinesis with mutism (stupor). *Journal of Mental Science*, **105**, 1088–94.

Starkstein S.E., Berthier M.L. & Leiguarda R. (1989) Psychic akinesia following bilateral pallidal lesions. *International Journal of Psychiatry in Medicine*, **19**, 155–64.

Steck H. (1926, 1927) Les syndromes extrapyramidaux dans les maladies mentales. *Archives Suisses de Neurologie et Psychiatrie*, **19**, 195–233, **20**, 92–136.

Steck H. (1931) Les syndromes mentaux post encephalitiques. *Archives Suisses de Neurologie et Psychiatrie*, **27**, 137–73.

Steck H. (1943) La conception Bleulerienne de la psychiatrie. *Annales Medico-Psychologiques*, **101**(1), 233–47.

Steck H. (1954) Le syndrome extrapyramidal et diencephalique au cours des traitements au largactil et ou serpasil. *Annales Medico-Psychologiques*, **112**, 737–43.

Stengel E. (1947) A clinical and psychological study of echo-reactions. *Journal of Mental Science*, **93**, 598–612.

Stevens J.R. (1973) An anatomy of schizophrenia? *Archives of General Psychiatry*, **29**, 177–89.

Stevens J.R. (1978a) Disturbances of ocular movements and blinking in schizophrenia. *Journal of Neurology, Neurosurgery, and Psychiatry*, **41**, 1024–30.

Stevens J.R. (1978b) Eye blink and schizophrenia: psychosis or tardive dyskinesia? *American Journal of Psychiatry*, **135**, 223–6.

Stevens J.R. (1982) The neuropathology of schizophrenia. *Psychological Medicine*, **12**, 695–700.

Stoddart W.H.B. (1926) *Mind and its Disorders. A Text-book for Students and Practitioners of Medicine*, 5th edn. H.K. Lewis: London.

Stone R.K., Alvarez W.F. & May J.E. (1988) Dyskinesia, antipsychotic drug exposure and risk factors in a developmentally disabled population. *Pharmacology, Biochemistry & Behaviour*, **29**, 45–51.

Straus E.W. & Griffith R.M. (1955) Pseudoreversibility of catatonic stupor. *American Journal of Psychiatry*, **111**, 680–5.

Symposium (1960) Extrapyramidal system and neuroleptics. *Revue Canadienne de Biologie*, **20**, 79–664.

Szabadi E., Bradshaw C.M. & Besson J.A.O. (1976) Elongation of pause time in speech: a simple, objective measure of motor retardation in depression. *British Journal of Psychiatry*, **129**, 592–7.

Taylor M.A. & Abrams R. (1973) The phenomenology of mania, a new look at some old patients. *Archives of General Psychiatry*, **29**, 520–2.

Taylor M.A. & Abrams R. (1977)   Catatonia, prevalence and importance in the manic phase of manic-depressive illness. *Archives of General Psychiatry*, **34**, 1223–5.

Teasdale J.D., Fogarty S.J. & Williams J.M.G. (1980)   Speech rate as a measure of short-term variation in depression. *British Journal of Social and Clinical Psychology*, **19**, 271–8.

Tourette G. de la (1985) Étude sur une affection nerveuse characterisee par de l'incoordination motrice accompagne d'echolalie et de coprolalie. *Archives de Neurologie*, **9**, 19–42, 158–200.

Tourette G. de la (1895)   *Traite Clinique et Therapeutique de l'Hysterie d'apres l'Enseignement de la Salpetriere.* Seconde partie. Plon, Nourrit et cie: Paris.

Trimble M. (1989)   Psychopathology and movement disorders: a new perspective on the Gilles de la Tourette syndrome. *Journal of Neurology, Neurosurgery and Psychiatry*, (suppl.), 90–5.

Turek I.S. (1975)   Drug-induced dyskinesia: reality or myth? *Diseases of the Nervous System*, **36**, 397–9.

Turner T.H. (1988)   Tardive dyskinesia. *British Medical Journal*, **296**, 719.

Tyrrell P. & Rossor M. (1988)   The association of gegenhalten in the upper limbs with dyspraxia. *Journal of Neurology, Neurosurgery and Psychiatry*, **51**, 995–7.

Udaka F., Yamao S., Nagata H., Nakamura S. & Kameyama M. (1984)   Pathologic laughing and crying treated with levodopa. *Archives of Neurology*, **41**, 1095–6.

Van Praag H.M., Korf J., Lakke J.P.W.F. & Schut T. (1975)   Dopamine metabolism in depressions, psychoses and Parkinson's disease: the problem of the specificity of biological variables in behaviour disorders. *Psychological Medicine*, **5**, 138–46.

Van Putten T., Mutalipassi L.R. & Malkin M.D. (1974)   Phenothiazine-induced decompensation. *Archives of General Psychiatry*, **30**, 102–5.

Verfaellie M. & Heilman K.N. (1987)   Response preparation and response inhibition after lesions of the medial frontal lobe. *Archives of Neurology*, **44**, 1265–71.

Vermeylen G. (1923)   Debilite motrice et deficience mentale. *Encephale*, **18**, 625–47.

Vermeylen G. (1938)   Les rapports cliniques entres les encephalites et la demence precoce. *Journal Belge de Neurologie et Psychiatrie*, **9**, 647–89.

Vrtunski P.B., Simpson D.M. & Meltzer H.Y. (1989)   Voluntary movement dysfunction in schizophrenics. *Biological Psychiatry*, **25**, 529–39.

Vujic V. (1952)   Larvate encephalitis and psychoneurosis. *Journal of Nervous and Mental Diseases*, **116**, 1051–64.

Waddington J.L. (1989)   Schizophrenia, affective psychoses, and other disorders treated with neuroleptic drugs: the enigma of tardive dyskinesia, its neurobiological determinants, and the conflict of paradigms. *International Review of Neurobiology*, **31**, 297–353.

Waddington J.L., Youssef H.A., Dolphin C. & Kinsella A. (1987) Cognitive dysfunction, negative symptoms, and tardive dyskinesia in schizophrenia. *Archives of General Psychiatry*, **44**, 907–12.

Waddington J.L., Brown K., O'Neill J., McKeon P. & Kinsella A. (1989) Cognitive impairment, clinical course and treatment history in outpatients with bipolar affective disorder: relationship to tardive dyskinesia. *Psychological Medicine*, **19**, 897–902.

Waddington J.L. & Youssef H.A. (1990) The lifetime outcome and involuntary movements of schizophrenia never treated with neuroleptic drugs. *British Journal of Psychiatry*, **156**, 106–8.

Walshe F.M.R. (1955) A clinical analysis of the paralysis agitans syndrome. In: M. Critchley (Ed.), *James Parkinson 1755–1824*, p. 245. Macmillan: London.

Watson R.T., Miller B.D. & Heilman K.M. (1978) Nonsensory neglect. *Annals of Neurology*, **3**, 505–8.

Webster D.D. (1968) Clinical analysis of the disability in Parkinson's disease. *Modern Treatment*, **5**, 257–82.

Webster K.E. (1975) Structure and function of the basal ganglia. *Proceedings of the Royal Society of Medicine*, **68**, 203–10.

Weckowicz T.E., Nutter R.W., Cruise D.G. & Yonge K.A. (1972) Speed in test performance in relation to depressive illness and age. *Canadian Psychiatric Association Journal*, **17**, 241–50.

Weiden P.J., Mann J.J., Haas G., Mattson M. & Frances A. (1987) Clinical non-recognition of neuroleptic-induced movement disorders: a cautionary study. *American Journal of Psychiatry*, **114**, 1148–53.

Weinberger D.R. & Kelly M.J. (1977) Catatonia and malignant syndrome: a possible complication of neuroleptic administration. *Journal of Nervous and Mental Disease*, **165**, 263–8.

Weiss B.L., Foster F.G., Reynolds C.F. & Kupfer D.J. (1974) Psychomotor activity in mania. *Archives of General Psychiatry*, **31**, 379–83.

White D.A.C. & Robins A.H. (1991) Catatonia: harbinger of the neuroleptic malignant syndrome. *British Journal of Psychiatry*, **158**, 419–21.

Widlocher D.J. (1983) Psychomotor retardation: clinical, theoretical, and psychometric aspects. *Psychiatric Clinics of North America*, **6**, 27–40.

Williams D. & Parsons-Smith G. (1951) Thalamic activity in stupor. *Brain*, **74**, 377–98.

Williams P. (1972) An unusual response to chlorpromazine therapy. *British Journal of Psychiatry*, **121**, 439–40.

Wilson S.A.K. (1912) Progressive lenticular degeneration. *Brain*, **34**, 295–509.

Wilson S.A.K. (1920) On decerebrate rigidity in man and the occurrence of tonic fits. *Brain*, **43**, 220–68.

Wilson S.A.K. (1925) Disorders of motility and of muscle tone, with special reference to the corpus striatum. *Lancet*, **ii**, 1–10.

Wilson S.A.K. (1927) The tics and allied conditions. *Journal of Neurology and Psychopathology*, **8**, 93–109.

Wilson S.A.K. (1931)   The approach to the study of hysteria. *The Journal of Neurology and Psychopathology*, **11**, 193–206.

Wilson S.A.K. (1940)   *Neurology*, Vol. 1. Edward Arnold: London.

Wimmer A. (1926)   Tonic eye fits (oculogyr crises) in chronic epidemic encephalitis. *Acta Psychiatrica et Neurologica*, **1**, 173–87.

Wing J. (1992)   Comment on institutionalism and schizophrenia 30 years on. *British Journal of Psychiatry*, **160**, 241–3.

Winkelman N.W. (1960)   The inter-relationship between the physiological and psychological etiologies of akathisia. *Revue Canadienne de Biologie*, **20**, 659–64.

Wolff E.A., Putnam F.W. & Post R.M. (1985)   Motor activity and affective illness. The relationship of amplitude and temporal distribution to changes in affective state. *Archives of General Psychiatry*, **42**, 288–94.

Woods B.T. & Short M.P. (1985)   Neurological dimensions of psychiatry. *Biological Psychiatry*, **20**, 192–8.

Wortis J. (1990)   The psychiatric literature: some perspectives. *Biological Psychiatry*, **28**, 1–2.

Wykes T. & Sturt E. (1986)   The measurement of social behaviour in psychiatric patients: an assessment of the reliability and validity of the SBS. *British Journal of Psychiatry*, **148**, 1–11.

Yahr M.D. (Ed.) (1976)   *The Basal Ganglia*. Raven Press: New York.

Yarden P.E. & Discipio W.J. (1971)   Abnormal movements and prognosis in schizophrenia. *American Journal of Psychiatry*, **128**, 317–23.

Yaryura-Tobias J.A. (1983)   *Obsesssive–Compulsive Disorders: Pathogenesis—Diagnosis—Treatment*. Marcel Dekker: New York.

Yazici O., Kantemir E., Tastaban Y., Ucok A. & Ozguroglu M. (1991) Spontaneous improvement of tardive dystonia during mania. *British Journal of Psychiatry*, **158**, 847–50.

Zametkin A.J., Stevens J.R. & Pittman R. (1979)   Ontogeny of spontaneous blinking and of habituation of the blink reflex. *Annals of Neurology*, **5**, 453–7.

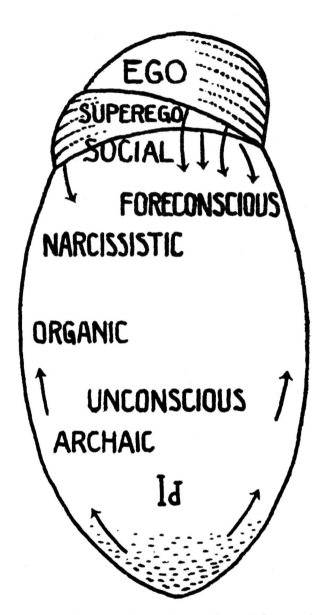

Figure 1 Investigation of abnormal mental states divorced from cerebral function: 'schematic diagram of mental apparatus' (modified from Freud), from Smith Ely Jelliffe's 1932 monograph on oculogyric crisis

(a)   (b)

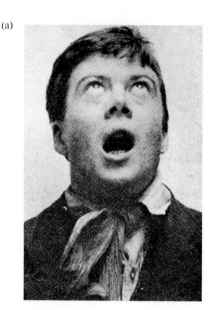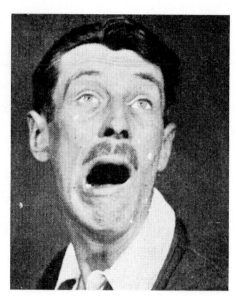

Figure 2 Psychiatry and neurology each with their own vocabulary for the same phenomena: (a) 'dementia praecox grimacing mannerism', from Norman's 1928 psychiatric textbook and (b) 'Post-encephalitic Parkinsonism with a mandibular tic', from Kinnier Wilson's 1940 neurology textbook. (a) Reproduced by permission of Churchill Livingstone; (b) by permission of Edward Arnold (Publishers) Limited

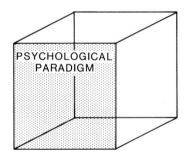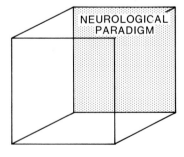

Figure 3 The Necker cube phenomenon—rival psychological and neurological paradigms for the same psychiatric phenomena. From Rogers 1988, by permission of Oxford University Press

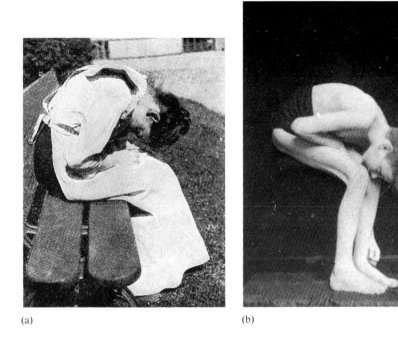

(a)   (b)

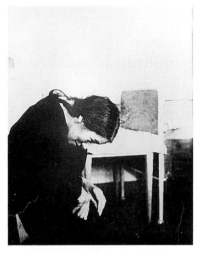

(c)

Figure 4 The same postural disorder in psychiatric and neurological disorder, from (a) Eugen Bleuler's chapter on schizophrenia in his 1923 *Textbook of Psychiatry*; (b) old photographs of post-encephalitic parkinsonism (Martin 1983) reproduced by permission of the *British Medical Journal*; and (c) an illustration of post-encephalitic parkinsonism with contractures in Hans Steck's 1926 thesis on extrapyramidal syndromes in psychiatric illnesses

(a)

(b)

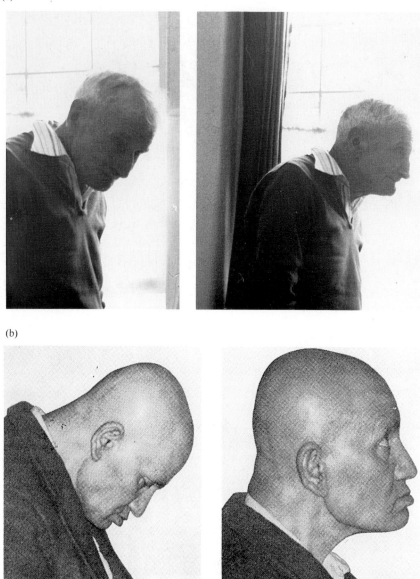

Figure 5 Reversible head flexion (left: usual position of the head; right: head raised by a voluntary movement) in (a) chronic schizophrenia (Rogers 1985), reproduced by permission of the Royal College of Psychiatrists; and (b) post-encephalitic parkinsonism (Martin *et al.* 1962), reproduced by permission of The Lancet Ltd

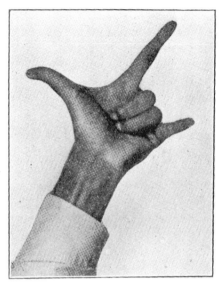
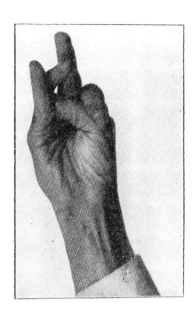

(a)

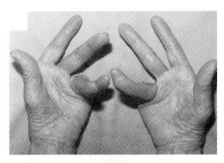
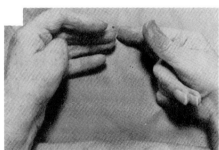

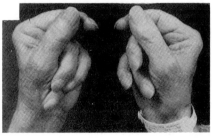

Figure 6 Abnormal finger postures from (a) Jelliffe and White's chapter on schizophrenia in their 1917 textbook of psychiatry and neurology, reproduced by permission; and (b) Kyriakides and Hewer's 1988 paper on hand contractures in Parkinson's disease, reproduced by permission of the *British Medical Journal*

(b)

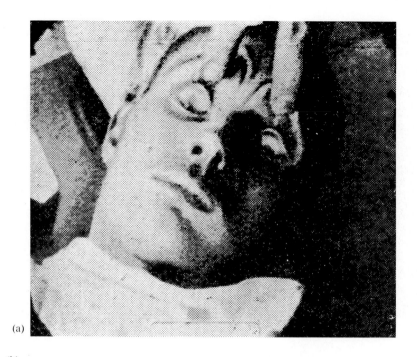

(a)

(b)

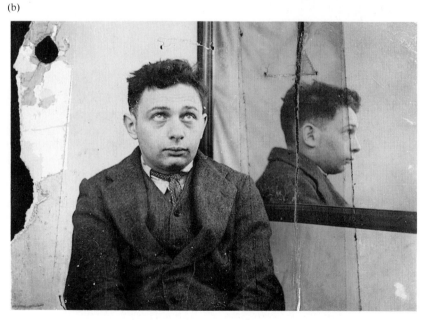

Figure 7 Oculogyric crisis in schizophrenia and encephalitis: (a) shows prolonged oculogyric spasm in a patient with hebephreno-catatonia reported by Paul Guiraud in 1936 reproduced by permission of Doin éditeurs, Paris; (b) shows the admission photograph in 1934 of one of the patients with chronic schizophrenia in the Friern study;

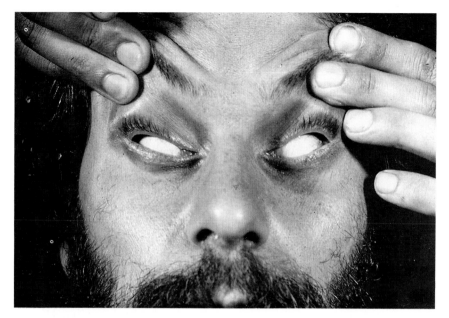

(c)

(d)

Figure 7 (*cont.*) (c) shows prolonged downward oculogyric spasm in a patient with catatonic schizophrenia in 1983; (d) shows downward post-encephalitic oculogyric crisis from Jelliffe's 1932 monograph

Index

Index compiled by John Gibson